SURVIVING WITHOUT YOUR MD

SURVIVING

WITHOUT YOUR MD

DO PRESCRIPTION DRUGS EVER CURE?

Eric & Glenna Edney

To order additional copies of this book, contact:
Xlibris Corporation
1-888-795-4274
www.Xlibris.com
Orders@Xlibris.com
66496

CONTENTS

CAUTION—DISCLAIMER

NOTHING IN THIS BOOK CAN BE GUARANTEED TO BE CORRECT. Of course, all that is said about our personal experiences and those of our family and friends are true. However, most anything else has been gathered from other sources. All we have done is gather information. We are unable to confirm all of the information from all the various sources. Most of the information seems to be correct based on our own personal experiences. We believe everything in this book is generally true and correct.

DEDICATION

This book is dedicated to a few of our friends whose skepticism convinced us to write this book. We realized that a few pages of written information would not prove our point of view. We gathered all of our information and put it in this book. The story is too unbelievable without the massive amount of information to prove it.

AUTHOR'S NOTE

A special note of thanks goes to several of our friends who were kind enough to read this book and make suggestions. That includes two medical doctors, two chiropractors, one dentist, one pastor, one nutritionist, one nurse, one proof reader, one TV personality and two ordinary people.

PREFACE

By Dr. Delos Soehren, D.C.

Today's fast paced "micro-wave" world has transformed our society into a "give me results NOW" mentality, but do we really know what we are asking for. When the average person has back pain or a headache, the typical course of action is to take some form of medication. Whether prescription or over-the-counter medication, it all has to be filtered through your liver and even prolonged use of something as innocuous as ibuprofen or aspirin can cause serious side affects. Even something like a vitamin-D supplement can have toxic levels, which can cause nerve damage, if taken in excessive doses.

Now consider one drug which was recalled in the largest prescription drug withdrawal in history. This recall was prompted by a new study that the drug caused an almost twofold increase in strokes and heart attacks. Ultimately, the drug killed approximately 140,000 people before the drug companies took it off the market. Now I ask you, how many people must die before a drug is determined to be unsafe? If the truth be told, there are NO safe drugs. Each and every one has varying degrees of undesirable side affects.

Now that I have your attention, you are about to be made aware of the "death-grip" that the drug companies have over the U.S.A. medical establishment. It has recently been determined that "medical care" is now the leading cause of death in the U.S.A. What? If you consider yourself an informed individual, then you owe it to yourself and your loved ones to find out what you can do to save yourself from the grips of the ever increasingly blatant disregard by the drug companies for "cures."

This book will cover many of these issues as well as give the reader several resources to help you stay away from pharmaceutical drugs, surgery and perhaps save your own life just like Eric did.

Dr. Delos Soehren
Clinic Director/Owner
Elite Health and Wellness, LLC
79245 Corporate Centre Drive, Suite 100
La Quinta, CA 92253
(760)771-5450 *Fax(760)771-5102
www.EliteHealthandWellnessLQ.com

CHAPTER 1

HEALTH CARE—WHAT I LEARNED THE HARD WAY

Having survived a TERMINAL ILLNESS for over eighteen years, I have learned a lot about health care in the U.S.A. Yes, that's exactly right; the doctor told me I had ALS (Amyotrophic Lateral Sclerosis a.k.a. Lou Gehrig's disease) and without the slightest doubt I would be dead in a few months. I had to learn a lot from that point on in order to save my own life. All that I have learned has created an irresistible desire to share the information with you and the whole world. This information could save your life. The problem is that my story is so UNBELIEVABLE that I must proceed slowly and provide you with a lot of information.

There are problems with our medical care system and we will review those problems in detail. During the process, we may be somewhat critical of our medical care system so be prepared.

When I say MEDICAL CARE SYSTEM, that means Medical Doctors, the AMA (American Medical Association), the Pharmaceutical companies, the government organizations such as the FDA (Food and Drug Administration), NIH (National Institute of Health), FTC (Federal Trade Commission) plus all the medical schools. When I use the term "health care system," that is all inclusive. The difference is that our problems are primarily with the medical doctors and the drug companies. The problems with our medical care system DO NOT involve other health care professionals such as chiropractors, nutritionists, and others who offer alternative treatments. I like all those people and I like all the personnel in the hospital ER.

Although the medical doctors are the front line of our medical care system, they are not the PRIMARY cause of our problems with the medical care system. There will be more on this later.

Before I launch into my campaign, it would be wise for me to tell you what some OTHERS have said about our system.

Earlier this year (2008), a retired high-level government official (I don't remember who) made this statement on national TV: *"Our medical care system is the MOST EXPENSIVE and the MOST INEFFICIENT in the whole world."* Now, that is saying a mouthful.

More currently, our own President Obama made the following statements in his talk before the AMA on Monday, 6-13-09: *"We are spending over $2 trillion a year on healthcare, almost 50% more per person than the next most costly nation."*

Perhaps of even greater significance he also said: *For all this spending, more of our citizens are uninsured, the quality of our care is often lower, and we aren't any healthier."* Now folks, this is important for you to know, so let me repeat AND WE AREN'T ANY HEALTHIER. How can anyone justify or explain all this expense and no benefit? Obama also said in referring to our health care system that it is a *"ticking time bomb."*

Let's look first at the COST of medical treatments.

Most of us already know that our medical care costs are high because medical insurance is high. In 2007, our total medical care cost was $2.2 trillion for an average per person cost of $7,421. If you are making a minimum wage and working 40 hours a week, your medical care cost will be approximately half of your gross income.

The average per person cost is more than double the average cost for people in other countries.

Our total medical care costs are 17% of our Gross National Product.

Again, the total medical care costs are well over $2 trillion every year; $2 trillion is 2 plus 12 zeros, and that's a whole bunch of money. Here is just one small part of that. In 2005, the total outpatient cost for prescription drugs was $200 billion. Congress recently passed a prescription drug bill that could add as much as $8 trillion to our total medical care costs.

The most unusual and alarming aspect of this problem is the relentless rate of increase year in and year out. Almost every year for many decades, medical care costs have increased at a faster rate than the general economy. In 2007, costs were up 6.1%.

Here are comparisons with two other countries:

1. In India, you can have major surgery for 10% or 15% of what it costs here in the U.S.A. and receive equal or better care.
2. Here is an even better indicator of high cost. It costs a Japanese company (Toyota) less than $300 per vehicle to provide medical insurance for its employees. It costs an American company (General Motors) over $1500 per vehicle. The Japanese company pays one-fifth or 20% of what the American company pays. To put it another way, General Motors has to pay over five times as much for medical insurance for its employees. That has a MAJOR effect on overall production costs and makes us less competitive with foreign companies.

Here is one more thought about costs. The cost of medical insurance is a major factor in most bankruptcy cases involving small and large companies plus individuals. The cost of all insurance is based primarily on the number of claims and the dollar amount of paid and reserved claims. The more sick people you have, the more claims you have. The more you pay out in claims, the more that raises the cost of medical insurance. So, don't blame the insurance companies as they are tightly controlled by the state insurance departments. They are not the cause of the problem.

Now, let's look at the INEFFICIENT part. When the retiring government official said INEFFICIENT, he did not elaborate. BUT, I think I know why he said that and that's what this book is all about. Let's look at some hard facts:

Evidently, we are among the SICKEST COUNTRIES IN THE WORLD. I read a few years ago that out of 125 countries in the world, we (the U.S.A.) are in last place. To say it another way, there are 124 countries where the people living there are healthier than we are. Now that one should make you wonder what's really going on. A few decades ago, the U.S.A. was among the top 10 healthiest countries in the world. The number of sick people has a direct effect on our medical costs. It's simple; the more sick people we have, the higher the costs. If we are among the sickest countries in the world and getting sicker, that MUST MEAN that we have an INEFFICIENT medical care system. I should be quick to point out that our medical care system is not the CAUSE of our health problems. Most of us follow an unhealthy diet and have insufficient exercise. There's much more that will follow later, but the main point here is that our medical care system is not properly equipped to handle our health problems. You will learn why I say that soon.

There are over 80 illnesses for which we have NO CURE. Oh yes, they have treatments, but no cure. Additionally, about half of our adult population has one or more chronic illnesses. Chronic means incurable. Now that's probably a lot more sick people than you ever thought. But the worse thing is that the list is getting longer, not shorter. Doesn't that make you wonder what's going on? Does all this sound like an inefficient system? I think so. You have probably been thinking, as I have, that we have the greatest medical care system in the world. Now, I don't think so anymore.

Here is another story that may cause you to question our medical care system. There is a clinic in Germany which has been doing stem cell transplants since 2007. In this country, we have been dragging our feet on stem cells for several years, due primarily to the moral or ethical controversy. BUT, the clinic in Germany uses the patient's own stem cells. They are removed from the bone marrow and moved to the desired location in the body. Using your own stem cells is the safest way to go as opposed to using someone else's stem cells and there's no morality issue. Now I ask you, why have we not been doing this? Also, why are we spending millions on stem cell research when Germany already has the answer? Why, oh why?

Here is another one. Michael Moore recently produced the movie called "Sicko." I'm not overly fond of Michael Moore because I find him a little abrasive. However, his documentary was factual and highly critical of our medical care system. One thought that stands out above all else in this documentary is this: Here in the U.S.A., we have a PROFIT-DRIVEN system. According to Michael Moore, there are three countries which have a NOT-FOR-PROFIT system; England, Canada and France. Coincidentally the people in all three of those countries live several years longer than we do here in the U.S.A. Give that some more thought. I think this is quite significant that people in three different countries live several years longer than we do. This is a clear indication that our PROFIT-DRIVEN SYSTEM is, in fact, inefficient.

The above stories may help you understand why our medical care costs are so high and also why our system is inefficient.

NEVER underestimate the POWER OF MONEY. I should say the love of money or greed. But the power of money sounds better.

THAT SHOULD BE A REAL EYE OPENER TO ANYONE READING THIS! Does that open your mind to the clear possibility that we have a problem? If you are the least bit open minded, then it should. I like to call myself an open-minded skeptic. I am skeptical of outlandish claims, but open minded to new ideas that are logical and probable. I LIKE LOGIC.

All of this is just the beginning. Hopefully this will open your mind to more information to follow. So, just sit back, fasten your seat belts and prepare yourself for a volume of evidence. The purpose of this book is not to find fault with anyone. The purpose is to inform you of the hazards in our medical care system. I say hazards because they will shorten your life unless you know about these pitfalls ahead of time. You will learn about the health hazards we all face and you will learn how to PREVENT ILLNESS and learn more about alternative treatments. You can and should live a longer, healthier and better life. You might be interested to know that wild animals have a life expectancy of two to one relative to humans. We should and could live much longer.

OK, we have now established the fact that we have a problem with our medical care system, but you may wonder how this all came about, or better yet, what set the stage for this to occur? The unbelievable part of this story is what people will do for a lot of money. It is amazing. To better understand this, we must first look at our history.

The problems with our medical care system were all PREDICTED OVER 200 YEARS AGO and by a MEDICAL DOCTOR.

Dr. Benjamin Rush was the only medical doctor to sign the U.S. Constitution in 1776. He signed it reluctantly because he had a firm conviction that we should have included more about MEDICAL FREEDOM. He was concerned that medicine would organize into an UNDERCOVER DICTATORSHIP. They could then limit both competition and new medical advances.

Here is one example of what he predicted would happen. This occurred about 75 years after the signing of the U.S. Constitution.

Looking back in history, here is the first example of exactly what he said would happen. Dr. Robert Barefoot tells the following story in his book "The Calcium Factor." It is just too good for me to paraphrase, so I will quote exactly what he said:

"In 1841 Ignas Semmelweis, a Hungarian physician who was horrified by the high death rate of women giving birth in hospitals, became obsessed with finding the cause of the disease. At that time mothers who had given birth at home or in carriages on their way to hospital had a far greater chance of surviving their childbirth than if they had been delivered in a hospital. Moreover, in that period it was common practice for doctors to go directly from the morgue, where they conducted post mortem examinations and anatomy classes using the bodies of deceased patients, into the maternity ward and attend maternity patients dressed in usual garb, without washing their hands. For these and other reasons, Dr. Semmelweis suspected that the doctors were carrying an agent on their hands

*that was causing the fatal disease. In 1847, Semmelweis instituted a procedure of scrubbing and dipping the hands in a chlorine solution before every procedure, the death rate fell from **thirty percent to practically zero**. The protective medical establishment of the day reacted by blocking Dr. Semmelweis's application for research funds and proceeded to vilify, ostracize, and finally have him discharged from his prestigious positions in maternity hospitals. Haunted by the fact that hundreds of thousands of women continued to die, Dr. Semmelweis eventually died of insanity in 1865."*

You may need to take a break from reading this book to actually digest and accept that story. It is so unbelievable to me. But, it is a matter of history and you can confirm it in the history books. You will notice that he uses the term "protective medical establishment of the day." Today, we call that the AMA (American Medical Association). What is the AMA and what do they do? It appears to me from their actions, that they are simply a "union" for the medical doctors. They appear to be more of a protector for the MD's.

You have not yet come to the real meat of this story, but I am sorely TEMPTED to provide you with a little foreshadowing of what's to come. Like one of my old girlfriends used to say, *"I can resist anything but TEMPTATION."* This will give you just an inkling of what I have learned about our medical care system.

The very first thing I learned of real significance from my ALS experience is that you should not believe EVERYTHING your medical doctor tells you. No one doctor can know everything about health care and all health treatments. That's why second opinions are more popular today. He may not be fully informed and he may not know that what he is telling you is wrong. However, that does not change the facts. This is especially true when a doctor tells you to go home and die, that there is nothing ANYONE can do for you. That may be true in some cases and not true in others. I have proven that to be untrue in my case. There are thousands more like me. I also know that it is not true when they tell you there is no known cure. There are no incurable diseases. There are many people alive today who have survived a so-called incurable disease. I am only one of them.

The Good Book says *"Seek and ye shall find."* Please note that it does not say seek and ye shall find except when your medical doctor tells you not to seek. There are no exceptions. How can you find anything if you don't look? Seek and ye shall find was written over 2000 years ago and is still true today, especially when you are looking for a cure for your illness.

If we lived in an ideal world, any good doctor would, upon diagnosis of an illness, provide the patient with more than one option. Currently, they simply don't do that. In most situations, they either give you a prescription for a drug or recommend surgery, as if to say there are no other options. That may not be the real truth. Actually, there are almost always other options. Here is just one example:

About two years ago, our daughter became very sick and went to the Emergency Room in severe pain in her stomach area. It took a couple of days, but they finally diagnosed the problem to be gallstones. They recommended immediate surgery to remove the gallbladder. Fortunately, we learned of a NATURAL treatment to eliminate gallstones. We found a web site on the Internet that explained in detail how to eliminate gallstones. The treatment takes less than 24 hours, you can do it in your home, it's very inexpensive, and very simple to do. Our daughter followed the instructions and passed many gallstones. THAT WAS THE END OF HER PROBLEM and without any expensive surgery. Doctors are all too quick to recommend surgery which may include a lifetime of problems following the surgery. The gallbladder is a necessary organ for good health. I have learned that removal of it may increase your chance of developing cancer and you will have a lifetime of digestive problems.

The gallstone removal treatment is also a liver cleanse. So I decided to try it for that purpose. Also, my wife, Glenna, has done it twice plus several of our friends have tried it. In every single case, we or they passed a large number of gallstones and the treatment worked perfectly.

I understand the doctors surgically remove about 50,000 gallbladders every year in the U.S.A. If each one costs $100,000, that would be $5 billion. Now that is a staggering figure. Think for just a minute about how much money we could save just by eliminating this one surgical treatment and substituting the natural treatment just discussed. Imagine the total savings if we could do more of that? Wow! Doesn't that just knock your socks off or what?

Here is the web site just in case you want it:
http://getridofgallstones.com/

Before we continue with more about our medical care system, you might be interested in knowing more about who I am. I'm the guy who saved himself from a 100% TERMINAL illness for which there is no cure or treatment. At least, that's what I've been told by the doctors.

Here is a little more about my story. My first diagnosis was in 1993. The doctor told me I had an untreatable and incurable illness. He said I had ALS (Amyotrophic Lateral Sclerosis) or Lou Gehrig's Disease. Now that in itself was a major shock. ALS is a living nightmare. The life expectancy is one to five years, but that is not the worst part. Here's what happens. You lose your strength and your muscles atrophy. That's bad, but it gets worse. In a short time, you have a normal mind with a normal libido living in a paralyzed body. Imagine that; a horny old man in a dead body (you 'gotta' laugh now and then). ALS is a living nightmare and the only escape is death (that is if you believe what they tell you).

The doctor told me to go home and put my affairs in order. In essence, he told me to go home and die! That seems impossible in this day and age. It just does not seem right for a doctor who has taken an oath to help patients with health problems to simply desert his patient in time of need.

I thought this simply cannot be and it just does not make sense here in the 20th century (1993). I always thought doctors were supposed to help you. Now they are offering me no help or even encouragement. They simply washed their hands of me. Doesn't that conflict with the Hippocratic Oath somehow? In 1996, the fourth doctor told me the exact same thing and that I would be dead before the end of 1997.

THE FIRST CLUE

All this experience gave me the FIRST CLUE that something may be wrong with our medical care system.

I accepted my fate for about two weeks. Then, my PMA (Positive Mental Attitude) stepped in and I decided NOT TO GIVE UP.

Eventually I learned that they were all wrong and that there was not only a treatment for my illness, but a possible CURE. I have had doctors tell me they could not help me several times before and I helped myself. I have cured myself of arthritis, asthma, psoriasis, back pain and IBS (Irritable Bowel Syndrome) all without help from any doctor or any prescription drugs. So I decided right then and there that I would beat this so-called terminal illness. Most of us are prone to accept and believe whatever our doctors tell us. But, if I would have believed MY DOCTOR, I would be dead now. Now that's a story in itself and I already wrote a book about that called "Eric is Winning." The purpose of this new book is to let you know what I learned about the many pitfalls in our medical care system.

THE SECOND CLUE

In 1996 I had my fourth and last diagnosis and then I began searching for answers. There are many of what I love to call "maverick" medical doctors and they write books. All in all, I've read over 30 books written by medical doctors and other health care professionals. That's how I learned what to do to save my life. Here I am being told by four different doctors that there's no treatment for my terminal illness, and yet there are other doctors telling me just the opposite. I judge this to be fairly convincing evidence that someone is not telling the truth. Actually, I did exactly what my doctors told me NOT TO DO. Instead, I followed the advice of the "maverick" doctors provided in their books. I believed them and they proved to be right. That means that the others must have been wrong. That was my SECOND CLUE that something was wrong.

THE THIRD CLUE

The THIRD CLUE came about two years later. The same doctor sent me a letter asking how I was doing. I thought that was very nice of him and I sent him a reply. I wrote a letter telling him a little bit about how I was doing, and more importantly, that I had stopped all progress of my ALS and actually had some improvement. I thought he would be interested in my experience. However, much to my surprise, he never answered my letter. Now I always thought that medical doctors learned from their patients. After all, they call their business A PRACTICE. In my mind, the word practice implies a learning experience. Wouldn't you think that he should be interested?

Here we have a medical doctor, a trained neurologist, and an ALS specialist who has a patient who is experiencing a miracle with a disease that has no treatment or cure and yet he had no interest in learning more about my experience. It has been my experience that most doctors rarely learn from their patients. It has also been my experience that no doctor has ever called me to learn the results of his prescription or recommendation. I realize this is the part that is hard to believe, but I will explain why that is happening later on in this book.

The mere fact that my "ALS specialist Loma Linda doctor" did not reply to my letter, TELLS ME A LOT. Oh yes, he received my letter. I called the nurse and confirmed that. She told me he would answer it, but he never did. They, or at least he, are not interested in learning anything about ALS. Why do they call him an ALS specialist and why would any doctor want to be an ALS specialist? What does an ALS specialist do to make him a specialist? Well, it appears to me that they don't do anything other than diagnosis. They make a lot of money doing diagnosis only and never have to recommend any treatment. Isn't that great? Really, I ask you, what are they offering their patients? What good is a diagnosis if there is no treatment?

If you are at all like me, you want to live life to the fullest, and to do that you must be healthy. So, what is your greatest asset? Is it your job, your home, your intelligence, your knowledge or your family? Actually, none of the above. You probably already know that your greatest asset is your health. Without your health everything else loses value and may be worth nothing.

The reason why I ask you that question is because the BIGGEST THREAT TO YOUR LIFE IS OUR MEDICAL CARE SYSTEM.

During the next several years, I learned much more about our medical system. If I told you all at once what I have learned, it would "stop your clock." So, I must proceed slowly and offer it in small doses. As the evidence piles up, you will begin to realize that it is overwhelming and undeniable that we have a major problem with our medical care system.

This will be hard to believe, but you must learn more about this. I only know that there is a massive amount of evidence that few people seem to know about. I've accumulated a tremendous amount of information about this problem that I wish to share with you.

CHAPTER 2

A LIFETIME OF EXPERIENCES WITH MEDICAL DOCTORS

Learning about our health care system began years ago for me.

Prior to my retirement, I spent almost 20 years as a salesman and before that several years in sales training both as a student and later as a teacher. All the sales techniques can be boiled down to two things. First, you must BELIEVE in yourself and your product or idea that you are selling. The second thing is very simple. If you truly believe in your product or idea, then you must have followed a logical thought-by-thought or step-by-step process to reach your conclusion. So, if you will take another person down that same step-by-step path, they should logically reach the same conclusion that you did. Doesn't that make sense?

Anyway, that's what I'm trying to do; that is to take you down the same path that led me to believe that we have a serious problem with our medical care system. It all started years ago. We will begin with all of my significant experiences with medical doctors throughout my lifetime.

I am 79 years old at the time of this writing. I have been to many different doctors for a variety of health problems during my lifetime. There is SOMETHING TO LEARN from each of my experiences, and you may find them interesting. These were my first learning experiences from my first doctor visit that I can recall up through my ALS diagnosis.

When I was about five years old, I ran two fingers of my left hand into the gears of a hand crank apple cider press. The doctor took good care of me that time except for the pain. Apparently the doctor thought that quickly tearing off the bandage was the best way to go. But he was wrong when the bandage is still attached to the scab on the wound. This was not a pleasant experience and I never forgot it.

*   *   *

During the ages of five to ten, I had measles and whooping cough and that's all. Although I was exposed to chicken pox by my next door playmate, I never had that.

*   *   *

I had many colds and runny noses when I was about nine or ten years old. My mother talked to three doctors about my problem and they offered no help. Finally, she found a good doctor. He asked my mother if I slept with my bedroom window open. She said yes. The doctor said to close the window at night. That was it; no more problems with colds. I tell you about that because if that happened today, the doctor would most certainly have given my mother a prescription for a drug. Most doctors just don't question the cause of a health problem.

Lesson: Not all doctors are equal.

*   *   *

At age ten, I developed asthma. Recently I read an article about chlorine and asthma/hay fever. These are two symptoms of the same problem. For the two years prior to that, I spent a lot of time in swimming pools with heavy chlorine. I used to ride my bicycle about three or four miles to the Bimini Baths and I swam there all day. They had three indoor pools and one of them heated. When you walked in, you were shocked by the odor of chlorine evaporating from the pools.

Eventually I outgrew the asthma/hay fever by the time I was about 19. It all came back when I was about age 28. The doctor said the trauma of a recent car accident and recent major surgery probably caused it to return. They don't have a cure for that. I simply lived with it for about 10 years. Then I ran across a book that suggested that comfrey root was good for asthma.

I bought some at the health food store and added some alfalfa to make it more palatable. I made one cup of tea and drank it every morning for about 10 years. Then, I realized I did not need it anymore. I have not needed it since. Before the comfrey root tea, I could tell you when I first walked into a house whether or not they had a dog or a cat. I would begin sneezing in less than two or three minutes. That is long gone. For the last 32 years I have lived with a dog and/or a cat inside our home with no problem.

Lesson: Asthma was cured with a natural treatment.

*   *   *

Psoriasis came along when I was about 26. It is a skin rash (non-infectious), and most doctors do not have a cure. Over the years, I've never had a doctor tell me what I had and I saw many doctors. Obviously, they did not tell me because they did not want me to know. They did not want to lose their patient by telling me it was incurable. I managed to cure many spots on my own and then I found one doctor who helped me cure a few more spots. I now have none. You would not know I ever had it. I bought a bottle of Siroil which contains tar. I would put the tar oil on my Psoriasis and sat out in the direct sun. I would apply the tar oil frequently during the day. I totally eliminated one spot in one day doing that AND that spot never returned.

Lesson: Another natural cure but with the help of a very exceptional doctor.

*   *   *

One of my most serious illnesses occurred at age 27. I developed Graves Disease; aka a toxic goiter. Simply put, I had an overactive thyroid. It was surgically removed with no problem. I had a great doctor and a great surgeon. But, here comes the interesting part. With no thyroid gland producing the natural thyroid hormone, you must take a thyroid supplement prescribed by the MD. Fortunately, my good doctor at the time prescribed the NATURAL hormone called Armour.

Now, I have moved around a lot over the years. Every time I move I find a new doctor for my thyroid prescription. EVERY TIME, without fail, the new doctor would order a new test before he will prescribe the thyroid. EVERY TIME the test is exactly the same. I have taken the same amount of thyroid for about 50 years. I don't mind the test too much, but here's what I really don't like. Every time the new doctor will prescribe the UNNATURAL drug replacement for my natural thyroid. I would always go along, but soon I would realize there is a difference. At that point, I would insist on going back to my NATURAL Armour thyroid.

Several years ago, I read an article written by a medical doctor. He made two points about thyroid:

One, there is no truly accurate test for thyroid. The best gauge is the PATIENT. If you take too much thyroid, you will be overly anxious, nervous and you will lose weight. If you take too little, you will become lethargic and gain weight. I know this to be true.

Two, the doctor also wrote that the natural thyroid hormone contains two known elements plus unknown elements. The DRUG thyroid contains only one element. Obviously, the natural Armour thyroid is much better. In spite of that, the medical doctor will always prescribe the drug thyroid if you let him. I don't.

Lesson: A natural substance is better than a drug.

* * *

For about ten years, from the ages of 35 to 45, I struggled with frequent anxiety attacks. There were times when I felt like my chest would explode. I learned after awhile that if I stood up and walked around, the problem would go away. The first time I went to a doctor about my problem, he gave me an EKG. That indicated no heart problem, so he simply wrote me a prescription for a drug to calm me down. I never had the prescription filled because I did not believe a drug was the answer. This doctor was younger than I at the time. He died two years later from a heart attack, so what did he know anyway? Nothing. Over the years I've had EKG's lying down, EKG's on the treadmill, and all for nothing. Finally one day at lunch I had an anxiety attack that was really scary.

I rushed right over to my doctor who tested me for everything possible. The only problem I had was high blood pressure. It was around 200/100. As you may know, that is stroke territory. He offered no help, but asked that I return in the early morning to have my blood pressure checked again. I did that and it was 120 over 77, which is quite normal. In thinking back, I remembered that I had a most anxious morning which started with a long, boring meeting during which I drank about six or seven cups of coffee on an empty stomach. Based on my experiences, I finally realized the answer to my problem with no help from any MD. I decided to quit drinking coffee and began jogging every morning before work. The problem has totally been eliminated and that was over 30 years ago. If that would have happened today, the doctors would have had me on many prescription drugs and I might not have lived as long as I have.

Lesson: Another natural cure.

*　　*　　*

One day as I was working at my desk, I had trouble focusing on the paper I was reading. I took off my prescription glasses and discovered I could read better without them. I have never had a pair of prescription glasses since then. I was about 45 then, and I'm now 79. You want to know what happened? A short time prior to that event I had began taking a high-quality multiple vitamin/mineral plus a B Complex 50.

Lesson: A natural vitamin does the trick.

*　　*　　*

Here is another story about my eyesight that occurred a few years later. I bought a pair of non-prescription drugstore reading glasses just so I could read the fine print in the stock listing in the newspaper. Then, a few weeks after I had been taking glyconutrients, I realized I did not need the reading glasses anymore. I could read the small print without them. Recently I had this same experience a second time. I had stopped taking the glyconutrients and my eyesight got worse. I began using my reading glasses everyday. Then, I began taking the glyconutrients and again my eyesight improved. I now use the reading glasses very seldom.

Lesson: Chalk up one more for nutritional supplements.

*　　*　　*

Here is one more recent eye problem. My left eye became bloodshot and I went to two different doctors. One said I had an infection; the other said no. However, they each gave me a prescription for eye drops (one cost over $100) and neither one of them worked. I tried Colloidal Silver and that helped more than either drug, but still my problem was not completely eliminated. Then, I remembered my mother always used boric acid for an eye wash. I use that now and then and it works better than anything else.

Lesson: Expensive drugs didn't help.

*   *   *

I first developed a prostate problem at about age 46. My doctor referred me to a prostate specialist. He recommended immediate surgery. I did not like him, so I sought a second opinion. The second doctor said I did not need surgery. My only symptom was I had to get up during the night to urinate. I decided I would rather live with that than have surgery. When I started taking vitamin E, my nighttime problem went away. Eighteen years later I finally had prostrate surgery to help urinate properly. Think about the value of a second opinion.

Lesson: You should not always believe the first doctor and never underestimate the power of money.

*   *   *

When I was about 48 years old, I developed extreme arthritis in my fingers and toes. One toe was so painful that it made me walk with a limp. The fingers were so painful it was very difficult for me to tie my necktie and I wore a tie to work five days a week. Some finger joints were painful, but others were completely frozen. I went to a doctor and he told me that I had arthritis and he painted a grim picture of what my future held. He offered no help at all. Then, we were talking to a friend's elderly mother who told me that tea bothered her arthritis. I realized that I had recently quit drinking coffee and switched to Lipton tea. Well, guess what? I quit drinking the tea and the arthritis in my fingers and toes went away and never came back. Now that is just too simple to be ignored. Why don't doctors know about that?

Lesson: One more natural cure.

*   *   *

You may find the next story very, very interesting. This one is about the cause of my ALS (Amyotrophic Lateral Sclerosis) and how I developed my terminal illness.

Like most PALS (Person with ALS), I was very active outside of work. I water-skied, hunted, fished and rode a dirt bike in the California deserts. I also jogged three miles every morning before work Monday through Friday. Glenna and I both played racquetball twice a week. I shot a 500-pound elk in Colorado and packed out half of it on my back in 1988. Of course, it took me two trips to carry out one-half of it. My two buddies carried out the other half. I was 59 years old then.

I also had an off-road race dune buggy. I didn't race it, but we used it for pleasure trips. Several friends of mine had them too. Four of the couples, including Glenna and I, planned a week long dune buggy trip in Baja California, Mexico in April of 1990. A few days before we were to leave, it looked like Glenna and I would not be able to make the trip. I don't remember why now but I'm sure it was work related. The other three couples left on the trip Thursday night. Late Friday, it looked like we could get away after all, but were we too late? We thought about it and then figured a way to catch up with the other couples.

The plan was to tow the buggies to Bahia de Los Angeles (Bay of L. A.), in Mexico, and drive the buggies from there. We knew that on the second night out of the Bay of L. A., which was Sunday night, our friends would be in San Ignacio. Because they would be traveling in sand washes and rugged dirt roads, we figured we could drive the dune buggy on the highway from the Bay of L. A. to San Ignacio and catch up with them. We knew this was a long shot. How would we find them in San Ignacio once we got there? We didn't know the answer to that one, but here's what happened. We were driving down the highway coming into San Ignacio and we had our CB radio on. Suddenly, we heard familiar voices speaking in English. Lo and behold, it was our friends headed out of town looking for a junkyard to find a replacement part for one of the buggies. I kept silent on the radio until they saw me. You can't believe their surprise.

Is this another example of PMA (Positive Mental Attitude) or what?

We had a great time on that trip! We continued on a big loop through all the back country of Baja and returned to the Bay of L. A. the following Saturday and Sunday we towed our buggies home. After we were home a few days, I developed chronic diarrhea. Well, that isn't unusual for having been to Mexico.

The stool testing in my case is a story all by itself. I went to my doctor and he suggested a stool test. After two weeks, I had to call the doctor to find out the results. She said the test proved negative, so they did not bother to call me. Since that did not solve my problem, I found another doctor. After three stool tests, by three different labs and no answer, I suspected a problem. So I called the testing laboratory and here's what I learned. The lab technician told me that it would take at least three or four separate tests to be sure of the results. I also had been given different instructions for caring for my stool samples. The lab technician told me·the right way to do it and I must tell you it was different from anything I had been told before.

Conclusion:

Most doctors don't know the correct instructions about stool testing.

Finally I learned the cause of my diarrhea. The actual name of the bug is Entamoeba Histolytica and it is as bad as the name sounds. If not treated properly, it is life threatening. The cure is terrible. They use a drug called Flagyl. Flagyl is a poison and highly toxic. It makes you so sick you can't believe that it is a cure. The only cure prior to Flagyl was arsenic. You had to take this poison to kill the bug and hopefully the bug would die before you did! You have probably guessed by now that medical doctors are not among my most favorite people. Well, here is one experience that will tell you why. I went to see four different medical doctors over a three-year period. Each doctor would recommend Flagyl, but the first three times it did not kill the bug. Then, now get this, I went to the Orange County Health Department (OCHD) and there I visited a doctor who really knew about Entamoeba Histolytica.

Here's what he told me:

Take 750 mg Flagyl three times a day for 10 days, and then

Take 650 mg Odoxin three times a day for 20 days.

These must be TAKEN IN SEQUENCE and never at the same time.

None of the other doctors had given me this precise formula. They had me take Flagyl alone or Flagyl and Odoxin at the same time. I went back to my last doctor with the information I had received from the *free service* at OCHD (Orange County Health Department). When I told my doctor what OCHD said, his reply was "It won't make any difference." Can you believe his arrogance? I said emphatically "I want to do it anyway. We must do something different from what we have done." I followed the Orange County formula and I got rid of the bug. How about that! The *amateur* wins again.

I started the above story with the buggy trip so you could see how close I came to avoiding all this. If I hadn't gone on the buggy trip, I might not have had dysentery, I wouldn't have taken Flagyl, and I might not have developed ALS. Oh well, that's life!

They say there is never anything so bad that there isn't some good in it. Perhaps you will see some humor in this story about my visit to OCHD. A friend had referred me to OCHD because another friend of his had a similar problem to mine and when his medical doctor couldn't help him, he found relief at OCHD. I called them for an appointment. After a long discussion, the lady on the phone said somewhat reluctantly, *"Well, come on in....I guess we will treat you."*

I didn't understand that at the time, but you'll understand in a minute. I arrived at OCHD and was directed to the waiting room. My first impression was the seriousness of everyone in there. This was certainly "Somber City!" After the usual wait, a man in a white coat called me into his office and began asking me a lot of questions such as *"With whom do you have sex?"* *"Do you have sex with women?"* *"Do you have sex with men?"* *"Do you have sex with both?"* Now there is an interesting question! I didn't understand all this, but I went along with it. Then he told me to wait in the waiting room again. Soon, I was ushered into another office to see "The Doctor." He began reviewing all the sex questions. At this point, my curiosity was overwhelming and I asked him *"Why all of the* **sex** *questions?"*

He replied *"You are in the VD Clinic!!!"*

Yes, VD as in Venereal Disease. I still didn't get it and I asked *"Am I in the wrong place?"* He laughed and said no. I asked *"Why am I being treated in the VD clinic?"* He said I had a sexually transmittable disease. I still didn't get it and I asked *"How do you figure that?"* He said *"Well you know how the guys do* it*."* Finally, the dawn came! It had never occurred to me that having amebic dysentery could be a sexually transmittable disease. Good thing they look at it that way, otherwise I might still have that Entamoeba Histolytica bug.

"Eric, what does all this have to do with ALS?" Well, it was shortly after this that I began to develop ALS symptoms. I believe ALS is caused by toxins. Flagyl is toxic. I believe taking Flagyl four different times was much more than anyone could normally handle without some serious adverse side effects. Also, many PALS (Person with ALS) have physical traumas related to the onset of ALS. I'm certain that this entire experience, including having diarrhea for three years, was traumatic to my system.

Here's another one on medical doctors. At this point in time, I still had diarrhea even though the Histolytica bug was gone. I asked my new doctor, I'm now on number five, what to do about my diarrhea. You won't believe what he said. He said *"Take Imodium anti-diarrheal caplets."* Well, I didn't take his advice because that sounded like a temporary solution to a long-term problem and incorrect. Instead, I found a nutritionist and colon hydro-therapist. She recommended an herbal pill. She suspected I still had some other bugs in there. I took the herbal pills as directed and my diarrhea stopped. What a relief!

Lesson: Recognize in the above story that the medical doctors did not cure my diarrhea but the alternative care person did cure it.

*   *   *

My first ALS symptoms occurred in 1990 with weakness in my right-hand grip. Then, a few months later, my right leg would not work normally and I began to trip. My first ALS diagnosis by a medical doctor was in late 1993. After all the tests were done and the diagnosis was in, I remember his nurse calling me to arrange another appointment. I recall asking her why the appointment? Could the doctor do anything to help me? She said no (of course). At that point I said, *"Well then, there won't be any need to make another appointment."*

I selected a doctor (Osteopath) who specialized in "alternative treatments" such as Chelation therapy and hyperbaric oxygen treatment. I enjoyed working with him. He's the one who later on told me I had to make my body as pure and ***pristine*** as possible by avoiding toxins. ***Pristine*** was a motivating word. THIS WAS BIG. That's what got me started on my program that led to my ALS protocol. When I first started with him around 1993, he didn't tell me to avoid any and all toxins. He did tell me to eliminate coffee and alcohol at that time, but I just couldn't do it. He did start me on a very comprehensive vitamin regimen. I was taking about ten or more vitamin tablets or capsules with each of three meals daily. The regimen included the following:

Vitamin E - 3600
Vitamin B1 - 300
Vitamin C - 500
Ginkgo Biloba
Mega Biotin - 7500 mcg
Sphingolin
Magnesium Oxide
Coenzyme Q10
B Complex - 50
Multivitamin
Pycnogenol - 100
Inositol - 3000 mg
Alpha-lipoic acid
Evening of Primrose oil
L-carnitine

In addition to the above vitamins, I had shots of Calcium EAP twice a week for about three months.

During this period from 1994 to 1995, my ALS symptoms were rather stable. I simply was not getting any worse. My right arm was partially paralyzed. My right ankle was stiff. Other than that, I was quite normal. I could walk all right except for the arthritis in my left hip. That caused me to use a cane. Talking, breathing, swallowing, and everything else were quite normal. I did not appreciate the fact that I was stable and not getting worse. Actually, that was quite an accomplishment, but I just did not realize it then. In retrospect, I should have realized that my condition had stabilized. However, I wasn't happy with just staying the same. I wanted improvement. When I didn't improve, I began to shortcut my vitamin regimen. In July of 1995, my left hip got so bad with arthritis I had to have a full hip replacement.

Now, here's where I find fault with another MD. I asked the doctor before the surgery if any of this would affect my ALS condition. He just shrugged it off and said *"We're only concerned with you living through the surgery."* *"Well, OK, you're the doctor."* I never want to say that again. I should not have trusted him; I should have pursued that much further. Immediately following the hip replacement in July of 1995, my ALS symptoms worsened. Up to that time, I only had limited motion in my right hand and arm and in my right foot. After the surgery, it moved into my left arm and left leg and my right leg got worse. They had given me morphine for pain in the hospital. They had also given me morphine to take home. I was taking the morphine off and on and after some time I realized that when I took the morphine, I was much weaker for one or two days afterwards. I immediately quit using the morphine and I quit having the relapses.

Lesson: All drugs are toxic and very damaging to a patient already suffering from an illness which is caused by toxins

*   *   *.

Although my ALS condition got a lot worse following the surgery, it remained stable through 1996. When I was diagnosed in 1993, the doctor said I had a motor neuron problem, but he didn't call it ALS. I know now that he thought it was ALS but couldn't tell me that. Since then, there have been three situations involving three different doctors who were reluctant to tell me I had ALS. They may not realize it, but I think they do you an injustice by not telling you. My first alternative treatment doctor never told me I had ALS. However, in a discussion with one of his nurses, she told me I had ALS. Now, how do you like that? The nurse tells you more than the doctor. Well, that's not the first time that happened.

My wife, Glenna, seeing my condition worsen following the 1995 surgery, finally convinced me to go for further diagnosis. I agreed. We considered all the major hospitals like UCLA, Scripps, and Loma Linda. We settled on Loma Linda. We first visited an MS specialist. After a very thorough physical exam, he referred me to the ALS specialist. The ALS doctor gave me an EMG, spinal tap, and bone marrow biopsy. All these tests were negative for other diseases and I had all the symptoms of ALS. Therefore, the conclusion is ALS. All my ALS symptoms included muscle weakness in my arms and legs, muscle atrophy, weight loss, slurred speech, fatigue and intense emotional responses to even the slightest situation.

Following these tests, I immediately began to deteriorate. My entire body got weaker. I began to choke on my food. My speech became slurred. In a very short time, I lost 15 pounds. That's a lot for my body weight. I started at 155 pounds.

These worsening symptoms and the ALS diagnosis are what really motivated me. I had a tremendous fear of ending up totally paralyzed, lying flat on my back, with nothing to do but think. That fear made me finally decide to go all out to beat this nightmare. That meant giving up my daily ration of Coors beer that I had enjoyed for around 40 years. It also meant no coffee, no ice cream and on and on; but I just had to do it. I decided to follow the advice given earlier by my "alternative treatment" doctor. That is, make your body as pure and pristine as possible! In other words, avoid ALL toxins.

I immediately put together what I will call my program. I was so convinced that my program would work that I wanted to write an article for the "ALS Digest." That's the e-mail newsletter that was published two or three times a week and e-mailed to over 5100+ PALS worldwide (PALS means a Person with ALS). I really wanted to share my ideas with the ALS world. However, my better judgement prevailed. I thought I had better wait until I've proven it before I write. I waited one year and after a great deal of improvement, I wrote my first article for the "ALS Digest."

Here is my program in a nutshell. In addition to PMA, my program has three parts or three steps:

Step 1—AVOID ALL TOXINS in your environment, especially in your home.

Step 2—Take all reasonable treatments to REMOVE TOXINS from the body.

Step 3—Provide the body with proper DIET and dietary SUPPLEMENTS. The main thing about the diet is that it should include more alkaline foods to raise the pH and it should all be ORGANIC.

Let me clarify something here. I believe we should look at the treatment of ALS as being in two phases:

Phase One—The object of Phase One is to **stop the progress of ALS.**

Phase Two—The object of Phase Two is to **restore the body** to its former condition.

Here is the basic idea in recognizing two phases. If your home was on fire, you would not start rebuilding your home until you first put out the fire. The same thing applies to treating ALS. One should have a lot of Phase

One treatments before progressing to Phase Two treatments. For example, any form of detoxification is a Phase One treatment. The controversial stem cell treatment is obviously a Phase Two treatment. It restores brain cells but does nothing to put out the fire. I believe you should know your objective before starting any treatment.

There is a lot of attention right now being focused on stem cell research. This could be a major breakthrough. However, I think it is a Phase Two treatment, not Phase One. Replacement of stem cells treats the symptom but not the cause.

Lesson: I treated myself with all natural treatments, no drugs and very little help from doctors (other than those who write books and my Chelation doctor).

*   *   *

There were two more problems soon after ALS; hip surgery and prostate surgery. They were both reasonably good experiences. No problems.

There is one more real lesson I learned from my ALS experience. I saved this for last because now we are getting down to the nitty-gritty.

*   *   *

This is an amazing story about my IBS (irritable bowel syndrome). After I had ALS for two or three years, I began to have bowel problems. This occurred long after I had eliminated the problem diarrhea that I picked up in Mexico. IBS is not a normal symptom of ALS according to the doctors, but I think it is. At any rate, I began to have diarrhea frequently. Every time I ate something the least bit out of the ordinary, I had a sudden occurrence and usually I would not get to the toilet soon enough. One day, Glenna and I were in Mammoth Lakes, California, and we stopped in a juice bar for a drink. I ordered a drink made primarily with carrots. Well, guess what happened? In less than thirty minutes, I had orange colored liquid flowing all down my pants and into my shoes and socks. Fortunately, I was able to get out of the car before that happened.

Do you know why drinking beer makes you urinate more frequently? Answer: Because it does not have to slow down to change color.

Well, the same thing applies to carrot juice I think. It does not have to slow down to change color either. OK, enough of that, let's get on with the IBS story.

This became such a serious problem that I began wearing a diaper 24 hours a day. I was making a trip to the bathroom three and four times everyday. One day I was in my doctor's office having a Chelation IV and I told him about my IBS problem. He wanted to put me in the hospital right then, I mean immediately. I did not go to the hospital. I came home and read a booklet on treating IBS with diet. That made sense to me rather than any drug or hospital. Here's what I did.

The very first thing they tell you is to go on a diet of white rice and yogurt exclusively for a minimum of three or four days. That means three meals a day of white rice and yogurt. When you have ALS, that means ORGANIC white rice (not brown—it won't work), and ORGANIC yogurt. Well, it wasn't fun, but it worked. Following that, I avoided all fruit and fruit drinks, all nuts, and any food the least bit spicy. Eventually, I had a lot of improvement, but I still would have one accident about every month. I believe that when you are going through detoxification treatments, you will have a problem about once a month because the body dumps accumulated toxins into your colon. When that happens, the body wants it out of there right now. That went on for a long time until I took chlorine dioxide. I must have had something like toxic pathogens in my colon because I had immediate improvement. My stools now are very solid most of the time and I just went 39 days without an accident. Even then, the accident could have been avoided because I ate something I should not have eaten.

One more thing about diarrhea that you may need to know. Cheese works really well. It will make your stool more solid. In fact, my great grandmother died from constipation from eating almost one whole pound of cheese in one afternoon. My diet now includes about two ounces of organic pomegranate juice twice a day, and I balance that with a chunk of organic cheese with breakfast and again with dinner.

Lesson: Most doctors would have written a prescription for my IBS in a heart beat. Again, I avoided a drug by using common sense and a natural cure.

OK, that is the end of the story about my ALS experience.

*   *   *

That brings us up to mid-year 2007 and I had a very interesting experience. I've had ALS for many years and I'm confined to a wheelchair for most the day. As a result of limited exercise, my legs began to swell. It became so serious that I went to the hospital. They were concerned about a possible blood clot moving from my legs to my lungs or heart and causing a serious problem. They put me on some drugs and after a few days, my legs were fine for the moment. They further recommended a drug that I would take everyday presumably for the rest of my life to prevent blood clots and leg swelling. The cost of the drug was about $2500 for a month's supply. I figured that was not the long-term answer.

I took the drug for one week and then switched to Nattokinase. Nattokinase is a dietary supplement made from the fermented soybean. The best Nattokinase is "Nattokinase NSK-SD." This is from the original enzyme discovered by a Japanese medical doctor.

The Japanese and Chinese are among the healthiest people on earth and they have eaten soybeans for centuries. Scientists attribute the soybean as a major factor. Based on my experience, I believe that what I have said about Natto is correct. It will simply dissolve and/or prevent blood clots. I have been taking Natto for a long time now and no problems with my legs swelling. If this product ever disappears from the market, you will know why. If everyone knew about how good Natto is, the drug companies would be very, very unhappy.

Lesson: Again, a natural cure beats expensive toxic drugs.

*   *   *

My next health problem occurred only a few months later. One morning I was leaning back to sit on the toilet when I just collapsed and fell down on the seat. Something happened to my back and I was unable to get up. The short story is that I sat there for three hours before finally deciding I just could not get up. Glenna called the ambulance and I was transported to the hospital. Here is where it gets really interesting. The ER doctor examined me and wanted to order several prescription drugs for me. I told him I would rather not do any drugs. He said that I was tying his hands behind his back; that he could do nothing for me and he went away. They did not want to admit me because I refused drugs. Can you believe that? After about a half hour the doctor returned and reluctantly agreed to admit me. Frankly, I was getting a little worried. I mean what do you do if they won't admit you?

After a couple of days of x-rays and other exams, I finally talked to a doctor who recommended an epidural. That's a one-time shot they inject right at the point of the problem. I agreed to do that because it was a one-time treatment. I absolutely refused to begin taking any drug that I might be forced to take the rest of my life. The epidural got me out of the hospital OK. Then I found a local chiropractor who has a computer-controlled decompression table. Here's the idea. Over the years we lose one or two inches of our height due to compression of the spinal column. Stretching the spinal column very gently allows improved circulation and re-growth. This is very expensive, but IT WORKS. I have had no problems now in over two years.

Lesson: Chiropractors are far better than drugs.

*　　*　　*

Now, for my last story in this chapter. This is the ONLY time I have been cured of any illness by medical doctors.

I had the hiccups one day for about eight or nine hours. I tried all the old remedies that had worked for me all my life, but they did not help. Finally, about 9:00 P.M., I gave up and went to the Emergency Room. I drove in on my three-wheel electric scooter. Two male nurses helped me stand up to transfer to the bed. They asked me first if I could stand. I said *"Yes, but with help."* Well, guess what, they helped me stand up and then turned loose of me. I began to fall and I pictured myself on the floor in about one second. BUT, they caught me before I hit the floor. Guess what happened? My hiccups were gone. I guess the fear of falling did it. I thanked them for the help and we went home.

Alright, you don't have to read anymore about my medical problems; this is the end of this chapter. Now for some medical stories about some other people.

CHAPTER 3

MEDICAL LESSONS FROM MY FAMILY AND FRIENDS

During my early years I learned a lot about doctors from the experiences of my friends and family.

Here is a story about my mother's health problem in 1943. I was 14 and this was the first medical experience that taught me a real lesson about MD's.

My mother became very sick and was placed in the hospital in Burbank, California. I was living with my dad in Beverly Hills. I rode my bicycle over 10 miles to see my mother in the hospital. I did not know at the time, but in those days they did not allow minors to visit patients in the hospital; not even their mother. Obviously, I was unhappy with the medical system. Hold on now, it gets really serious and much worse. The doctor told my stepdad that my mother had a serious infection in one kidney. The doctor recommended surgery to remove it. My stepdad said no, and took my mother out of the hospital over the doctor's objection. My mother went to another doctor who cured her and she remained problem free for many years. She had another flare-up with the kidney about 1965, over 20 years later. During that hospital visit, my mother learned for the first time that she had only one kidney. Wow, imagine that. If the first doctor would have had his way, my mother would have died in 1943. That experience taught me a lot about doctors.

Lesson: Always consider a second opinion and never underestimate the power of money.

*   *   *

I can hardly believe this happened. It was a real shocker. Here it is in late August 2008 and while I'm in the middle of writing this book, another close friend died. Gary was my friend of over forty years and one of my desert motorcycle riding companions for most of those years. We did not even know he was sick and in the hospital. We received a phone call on Sunday, August 24 about 11:00 A.M. We learned that he went into the hospital 10 days earlier for fairly minor surgery. We were also told that he was in very serious condition and the situation was not good. He died at 3:00 P.M. that same day.

Now, here's what's hard to accept. HE DIED OF AN INFECTION that he did not have before he went to the hospital. Can you believe that?

About 90,000 people die every year from infections that they get in the hospital. Now I see two problems with that:

#1 The hospital provides the environment to give the patient the infection.

#2 They evidently are unable to treat it even though the patient is already in the hospital and they know the problem.

Evidently antibiotic drugs are becoming far less effective than they were years ago and that's true of even penicillin. There are better antibiotics available. One of them is chlorine dioxide (more on that later). I believe that could have saved Gary's life.

What is really hard to accept is that Gary was a very healthy and very active man. There must be some reason why this is happening. It does not seem reasonable that a healthy man can be very much alive one day and then 10 days later he's dead from something so simple. I thought our medical system was far better than that. Here is one possible explanation: Gary was taking a few prescription drugs. There are some drugs which can impair the immune system and reduce the body's ability to fight infection. The drug makers may warn you about this, but they don't actually say that this may be fatal. They rarely say that about their drugs, although hundreds of thousands die every year from toxic prescription drugs. I don't know about you, but that really makes me question the integrity of our medical system.

There is no proof that Gary died of a drug. It is very difficult to prove that in any case. I believe the drug companies know this all too well and rely on this fact.

Now I have read that about 90,000 die from infection while in the hospital, but when a person really close to you dies, that's a horse of another color. Gary was my wife's ex-husband. Well that's really close to home. It may be hard for some to understand, but Gary and I, as well as Glenna and Gary, remained close friends for all these many years. In fact, Glenna and I both attended the funeral and Glenna had a major role in the service.

A couple of months after Gary died, we had a conversation with his widow about him being in such good health before his passing. She said *"Gary put too much TRUST in the doctors."*

Lesson: Hospitals are dangerous; avoid them if you can.

*   *   *

My mother's aunt developed psoriasis way back around 1920, long before any drug company's influence. Her doctor was able to completely eliminate all of the skin lesions with a combination of diet and Epsom salt baths. Also, she would lie out in the sun immediately after the Epsom salt baths.

Lesson: Natural is good.

*   *   *

My friend's father was born in Mexico and my friend brought her father to this country several years ago. Naturally, that changed his diet a lot and he developed intestinal problems. The doctor prescribed a drug which soon began causing side effects, so the doctor prescribed another drug. Soon he was taking seven different drugs! After about two years on these drugs, they told him his problem was incurable and he had only six months to live. My friend and her father decided there was no point in continuing all those drugs as he would die anyway. So he quit taking the drugs and returned to his home town in Mexico to die. Well, he did not die in six months as they told him he would. He died all right, but nine years later at the age of 95!

Lesson: Many times the drugs are the cause of your illness.

*   *   *

Glenna's stepdad developed a back problem. I suggested that he see a chiropractor. He did not do that and opted for back surgery. It is now five years after the surgery and his back is worse than ever. I have never known anyone who has experienced improvement from back surgery.

Lesson: Consider a chiropractor before back surgery. It is more natural.

*   *   *

My Uncle Harvey developed a really serious skin problem. His skin turned a dark purple color all over his body and was scaling a lot. His skin was so dry, it would crack and bleed. He went to several doctors but with no avail. My parents had recently purchased a 40 acre plot of land near Mammoth Lakes, California which included a natural hot springs. My stepdad was quite clever and piped in the natural hot mineral water to a bath tub in their home. They invited Uncle Harvey to come up and try soaking in the hot springs mineral water. Harvey soaked in the tub one hour everyday for about a month. Finally, one night when Harvey was soaking, he hollered out for my stepdad, George. George rushed in and found black liquid flowing from Harvey's leg and a golf ball size lump that had fallen out of his leg leaving a large hole. After a couple of minutes, the bleeding turned red. From that day on, Harvey's improvement was better and better. He was totally cured after about three months.

No one knows the real cause of his problem, but we are guessing that he must have been bitten by a toxic spider or some other insect.

Lesson: Another cure by a natural treatment that some people might not believe.

*   *   *

My stepdad, George, had a terrific back problem when he was about 40 years old. One morning it was so painful he stayed in bed and could not go to work. During that day, the pain became so unbearable that he struggled out of the house and into his car. He drove to the first medical doctor he could find and went in. He told the doctor he just wanted something for the pain. The doctor gave him a shot and his pain lessened immediately. He returned to the doctor frequently and had remarkable improvement over the next month. Then one day he asked the nurse *"What in the world is in the shot?"* The nurse replied *"Vitamin B-1."* This all occurred when George was about 40 years old. He continued to take vitamin B-1 orally the rest of his life and never had another back problem. He died at age 78.

Lesson: One more natural cure.

*   *   *

During my lifetime, I've seen a lot of people die from cancer. Most of them have chemotherapy treatments and I know of no one who benefited from it. It appears to me that the chemo just makes the last days of their life worse. I decided a long time ago that I will never do chemo. But more than that, I have learned recently that there are many possible cures for cancer and there's no need for chemo treatments.

Over the years, several of my high school buddies have kept in touch. About five years ago, five of us began an annual get-together; Al, Eric Peacock, Bruce, John and myself. I mention this to let you know that these are all close friends of mine. About one year ago, I heard from John that Eric had cancer. I immediately mailed him a letter with all the cancer information I had and warned him about the dangers of chemotherapy. Eric called me immediately to let me know that he was doing just fine and had already started on the chemotherapy. He was having no problems with his chemo treatment. Well, what can you say? I sent him all the information and he just ignored it. (This story is a lead-in to the next chapter). So, I said no more. One week later Eric was out hunting with a friend. Eric shot one quail and collapsed. When his friend got to him, Eric was already dead. This was no doubt caused by the chemo. One possible side effect of chemotherapy is an aneurysm where the artery bursts and when this happens your blood pressure drops dangerously low. About 90% of all aneurysms are fatal.

You may not know it, but it is so frustrating to know what I know about health and not be able to prevent things like Eric's death. I truly believe I could have saved Eric's life with what I know and that is so frustrating.

Lesson: Learn about alternatives and learn about the risks of chemotherapy before any treatment.

*   *   *

This story is about our friend Paul. This is a good story and that's why I saved it for last in this chapter.

About a year and a half ago, Paul was diagnosed with Polycythemia. You may not know what that is so let me tell you. Apparently it is simply a condition where your blood gets really thick and turns to sludge. Obviously, that is life threatening. As I understand it, they have no cure and the only treatment is Phlebotomy or chemotherapy. Phlebotomy simply means draining some blood out to thin the blood. I thought that was a medieval treatment they gave up a hundred years ago. Apparently not. Again, the medical doctors have no cure and they evidently do not have a clue about the cause.

I provided Paul with an article written by medical doctors about excess iron in the blood possibly being the cause of Polycythemia. Paul was also aware of the supplement Nattokinase. The following is what Paul did and his results. Originally Paul was having two pints of his blood drawn every week. Then he began a diet of eliminating all foods with any iron such as red meat, red wine, and dark green vegetables. He also began taking one capsule of Nattokinase a day.

Here are the results of his blood draw:

Two pints a week for one month.
One pint a week for two months.
One pint every two weeks.
One pint a month.
One pint every three or four months.
Imagine that, all this improvement with no drugs.

Conclusion

I don't think any of these stories are isolated cases. I think these things happen everyday all over America.

MY EXPERIENCE OVER THE YEARS HAS TAUGHT ME TO BELIEVE THAT NO ILLNESS IS INCURABLE.

CHAPTER 4

LIST OF BOOKS

Most medical doctors practice only what they have been taught in medical school. Medical schools teach almost nothing about toxins or nutrition. There are a few doctors who have realized after years of practice that they are unable to cure many of their patients. Some of these WONDER doctors are my heroes because they write books about what they have learned. I've been in a wheelchair for way over ten years because of a prescription drug. My health problem could have been treated another way rather than the drug, but that's all most doctors treat their patients with and I was no exception. Now you might question whether or not these doctors who write books are correct or not? Well, in my opinion, they are and let me tell you why I say that. First, reading their books is what saved my life when the regular MD's could not. Secondly, I don't think doctors write books about health to make a lot of money and that's putting it mildly. Thirdly, the MD's who write these books are putting their professional status on the line by disagreeing with mainstream thinking. I believe they are writing these books with a sincere desire to help people who are not being helped by mainstream MD's.

The following is a list of books which I have read. I believe they were instrumental in helping me. I'm not suggesting that you read them all, but of course that would not be a bad idea if you are interested in your health. The main reason I list them is so you can see who is writing them and the SUBJECT of the book. Also, I have made remarks about each book.

There may be a hundred or more books of this type and I'm only listing a few. The people who write these books are either lunatics or they are right. If they are right, then we have a huge problem with our entire medical care system. Do you think they are right or not? You might want to keep that question in mind while you continue reading this book. You may find the answer.

Here is the list:

"World's Greatest Treasury of Health Secrets" by medical editor Arthur P. Johnson. This is actually an accumulation of several hundred medical doctors.
You may order this book from:
https://www.bottomlinesecrets.com/store/books/order_hsuc.html?sid=store

"Natural Cures 'They' Don't Want You to Know About" by Kevin Trudeau

The above two books are listed first because they both provide you with many NATURAL CURES and they both provide much evidence about the problems with our medical care system. You might want to read them. These two books plus the one you are reading would be good reference books for you in the future.

"The Calcium Factor: the Scientific Secret of Health and Youth" by Robert R. Barefoot & Carl J. Reich, MD.
This is one of the first books I read after my ALS diagnosis and you will find this one very interesting.

"Forty Something Forever, a Consumer's Guide to Chelation Therapy and other Heart-Savers" by Harold & Arline Brecher.
This one provides a lot of good information about your heart.

"The pH Miracle—Balance Your Diet, Reclaim Your Health" by Robert O. Young, Ph.D., and Shelley Redford Young.
Here is a MUST READ book.

"Cancer Doesn't Scare Me Anymore" by Dr. Lorraine Day.
This is not a book, but rather a video tape. However, Dr. Day has written some books.

"The Grape Cure" by Johanna Brandt from The American School of Naturopathy.

This book was written almost one hundred years ago and all about curing cancer and other diseases.

"Self-Treatment for AIDS, Oxygen Therapies, Etc." edited by Betsy Russell-Manning.

This book is also about treating cancer.

"The Gerson Therapy" by Charlotte Gerson and Morton Walker, D.P.M.

Another one about treating cancer.

"How to Fight Cancer & Win" by William L. Fischer.

And still another one.

"German Cancer Breakthrough" by Andrew Scholberg.

Here is one more.

"Medication Madness" by Peter R. Breggin, MD.

"Brain-Disabling Treatments in Psychiatry" by Peter R. Breggin, MD.

"Toxic Psychiatry" by Peter R. Breggin, MD.

The above three books are all about drugs and mental health.

"Detoxify or Die" by Sherry Rogers, MD.

"Alkalize or Die" by Dr. Theodore A. Baroody.

The titles of the above two books speak for themselves. These are must read books.

"There Are No Incurable Diseases" by Dr. Richard Schulz.

Here is another must read.

"The Cure—The 12-Week Plan to Prevent and Reverse Cancer, Heart Disease, Obesity and More" by Dr. Timothy Brantley.

Here is still one more book on treating cancer.

"Excitotoxins: The Taste That Kills" by Russell L. Blaylock, MD.

"In Bad Taste, The MSG Syndrome" by George Schwartz, MD.

The above two books should convince you of the truth about how toxic MSG and Aspartame are.

"The Cure for all Diseases" by Hulda Regehr Clark, Ph.D., N.D.
Here is a fantastic book written by a very unusual and well-credited doctor. The book includes many actual patient case histories. The following quote is taken right from the cover of the book: "New research findings show that all diseases have simple explanations and cures once their true cause is known. This book describes the causes of both common and extraordinary diseases and gives specific instructions for their cure."

"It's all in your Head—The link between mercury amalgams and illness" by Dr. Hal A. Huggins. *Yes !! I agree / I was poisoned*
There are over forty books linking dentistry, especial Mercury amalgams, and illness. This is my recommendation for the book you should read first.

Again, you must ask yourself are the authors of these books really nuts or are they giving you solid advice? Now I know the answer to that, but do you? I believe these books are solid evidence that we have a serious problem on our hands in our medical care system.

SINCE MOST OF THESE BOOKS WERE WRITTEN BY MEDICAL DOCTORS, DON'T YOU THINK IT WOULD BE A GOOD IDEA IF ALL OF THE OTHER MD'S READ THEM? I don't think they do.

CHAPTER 5

THE NOBEL PRIZE IN MEDICINE

A brief review of all the Nobel Prize winners in Medicine has revealed some very interesting information. A Nobel Prize in Medicine has been awarded to one or more doctors in almost every year beginning in 1901. They only missed a few years during World War I and again in World War II. The following list includes only the Nobel Prize awards in Medicine which are all obviously for some discovery which led to a cure or successful treatment. There are twelve awards which are ALL for infectious diseases except for one in 1931. That one did not lead to a cure but it should have. What's really interesting to me is that our medical system has only recognized the cures for infectious diseases and ignored all others. Since 1955 there have only been two more awards that appear to be for a cure: 1998 and 2007. These three awards, 1931, 1998 and 2007 have all been totally ignored. I wonder why? You might be interested to know that all three of these discoveries are in use today but only in other countries; not here in the U.S.A. Again, I wonder why?

1901—Emil Adolf von Behring—for his work on serum therapy and diphtheria. This led to a victory over diphtheria.

1902—Ronald Ross—for his work on malaria and successful methods of combating it.

1903—Niels Ryberg Finsen—for his contribution to the treatment of diseases, especially lupus vulgaris.

1905—Robert Koch—discoveries in treating tuberculosis.

1907—Charles Louis Alphonse Laveran—for his work in successful treatment of infectious diseases.

1923—Frederick Grant Banting and John James Richard Macleod—discovery of insulin.

1927—Julius Wagner-Jauregg—discovery in the treatment of dementia paralytica (malaria inoculation).

1931—Otto Heinrich Warburg—discovery of the nature and mode of action of the respiratory enzyme. This also included the discovery that a cancerous tumor was anaerobic (living without oxygen).

1945—Sir Alexander Fleming and Ernst Boris Chain and Sir Howard Walter Florey—discovery of PENICILLIN and its curative effect in various infectious diseases.

1951—Max Theiler—discoveries concerning yellow fever and how to combat it.

1952—Selman Abraham Waksman—discovery of streptomycin, the first antibiotic effective against tuberculosis.

1954—John Franklin Enders and Thomas Huckle Weller and Frederick Chapman Robbins—discovery of the ability of POLIOMYELITIS viruses to grow in cultures of various types of tissue.

1998—Robert F. Furchgott and Louis J. Ignarro and Ferid Murad—discoveries concerning nitric oxide as a signaling molecule in the CARDIOVASCULAR system.

2007—Mario R. Capecchi and Sir Martin J. Evans and Oliver Smithies—discoveries of principles for introducing specific gene modifications in mice by the use of EMBRYONIC STEM CELLS.

CHAPTER 6

CANCER

It is time to again warn you that I am only a reporter but with an opinion; all I do is gather information from what I believe to be credible sources. I cannot guarantee that everything I say in this book is true. I believe it's true or I would not report it.

Cancer is expected to overtake heart disease to become the number one cause of death worldwide by 2010, according to the World Health Organization (WHO).

Not long ago, I realized that I have not only learned how to prevent illness but also how to successfully treat most any illness. Yes, even cancer and heart disease.

If I told you that I knew of a cure for cancer, you would either laugh or think that I am completely insane or just drank too much "red goofy" (wine). You probably think that we have the greatest medical care system in the world and, if there was a cure for cancer, your medical doctor would know all about it. The whole purpose of this book is to encourage you to question whether or not that is really true. Now I am no health care professional or an expert on health treatments. I am fairly intelligent and have a good memory. I simply gather information. Here is the information I have gathered about cancer.

Before we go any further on cancer, let me ask you one question. Do you think it's LOGICAL that today, in the 21st century when we have put men on the moon, that there is no cure for cancer? Now, you must think about that a minute and realize that we already know the cause. Knowing the cause is half the battle in problem solving. My common sense tells me that we should know a cure.

What do we really know about cancer? I THINK we know quite a lot. I may be wrong, but based on what I've read, the following is possibly true:

We know it's anaerobic

That means living without oxygen.

We know more sunshine means less cancer

Studies have proven that sunshine on our bodies causes the body to produce vitamin D, which in turn contributes to the prevention of cancer. Less sunshine means more cancer. Why do doctors always tell us to stay out of the sun?

We know more Selenium means less cancer

People living in areas where the soil has low Selenium have more cancer.

We know that carcinogens can cause cancer

We also know that carcinogens are first toxins. There is a high probability that any toxin may cause cancer. Curing almost any illness becomes relatively simple when we already know the cause. To know the cause is to know the cure.

We know certain foods can prevent cancer

Cruciferous vegetables, asparagus, Ginseng, mushrooms, Sterols and Sterolins. Also onion and garlic (garlic contains Selenium). Note: This is not all, but just a few examples.

We know that cancer loves sugar

According to almost all nutritionists, sugar should be avoided as much as possible. Some recommend Stevia instead.

We know certain foods can cause cancer

Avoid margarine—real butter is better. A Harvard research study concluded that cancer was linked to the consumption of margarine, hydrogenated oils and shortenings.

Avoid non-organic food—Normal commercially grown produce contains toxic heavy metals. Children receive up to 35% of their entire lifetime supply of pesticides by the age of 5. Trace amounts of 17 pesticides were found in baby food sold in the U.S.

*   *   *

TV documentary—"The Unexplained"

This story should cast serious doubt that THERE ARE NO CURES FOR CANCER. This story is from a TV documentary on the Biography channel aired on 4-27-08 (first aired 1-28-99). This story is about 59 year old Jean Reinert who was a life long smoker and who developed lung cancer. The story begins 9-1-94 when Jean had malignant lung cancer which had spread to her esophagus and with a large tumor touching her heart. The doctor said it was inoperable and gave her six months to live. Only one in eight women survive lung cancer even if caught early.

Jean did not believe her doctor and found Block Medical Center and Keith I. Block, MD and founder of the Block Foundation for Medical and Nutritional Research. He was a cancer specialist from the University of Illinois. His cancer therapy included both conventional and unconventional therapy including Chinese herbs, exercise, and macrobiotic diet. His conventional treatments included 12 radiation treatments. Jean had no side effects which are normally expected with radiation. One month after the original diagnosis, her tumor was almost gone.

Later on during more testing, they discovered the cancer had spread to her brain. More radiation, exercise and diet. By the end of November, the brain tumor was gone.

Then, wouldn't you know it, in a routine check up, they discovered cancer in her spleen, neck, right kidney, her right adrenal gland, lymph nodes, and abdomen. At this point, most doctors would throw in the towel, but not Dr. Block. He started Jean on chemo, adjusted her diet, and added a compound of Chinese herbs to boost the immune system.

In March, six months after being told she only had six months to live, her cancer was completely gone. She remained on the diet and as of 1999 was still cancer free.

Now, I simply must add my comments here. This is an unbelievable story, but well documented with all the names. This doctor not only successfully treated Jean for cancer, but he did it THREE TIMES. This story seems to indicate that there are cancer cures other than what the doctors normally offer which is chemo, radiation and surgery only.

The doctor in the above story may never become rich or famous even though he may have developed a better treatment for cancer. The system is anti-cure. This story is now ten years old. Have you heard of any changes in our treatment of cancer based on this story? No, and you never will in my opinion.

Will all doctors ever have a cure for cancer?

You probably answered yes. Sooner or later they must find a cure. It is not logical that no cure exists now or ever will exist.

Will it be the drug companies who develop the cure?

Answer: Let's try a little more logic again. Each person who is newly diagnosed with cancer is worth over $300,000 to the medical system. About 1.5 million people in the U.S. alone are newly diagnosed with cancer each year. Multiply that out and you have $45 billion. THAT'S THE TOTAL VALUE OF ALL CANCER PATIENTS TO OUR MEDICAL CARE SYSTEM. You might look at it this way; cancer is the golden goose that lays the golden eggs. If we developed a cure for all cancer, the income to the medical care system in the U.S. would be reduced by $45 billion.

I have trouble contemplating just how much money that really is. So, let's compare that to one of the largest corporations in America—Bank of America. That amount of money could buy over half of all outstanding shares of Bank of America at its present price of about $12 per share. A couple of months ago you could have bought it all. Now, you should realize that is a shocking amount of money.

Do you think for one minute that THEY want to find a cure and put themselves out of business and out of work?

Never underestimate the power of money.

There was a one-hour television program called "Stand Up to Cancer" that was broadcast on three networks at 8:00 PM on 9-5-08 for the purpose of raising money for more cancer research. Among other dollar figures on the cost of cancer, they stated the following:

A 1% REDUCTION IN THE NUMBER OF DEATHS FROM CANCER WOULD ADD $500 BILLION TO THE U.S. ECONOMY.

I don't know how they figure that, or how it relates to the $45 billion. Nonetheless, that's what they said.

I know that's extremely difficult to "get your head around," but those are the simple facts. You may draw any conclusion you want.

We already know, and it's a matter of "record," that the tobacco companies lied to us about the hazards of smoking tobacco. Why did they lie? The answer is "To protect their income."

Never underestimate the power of money.

Here are some indisputable facts all relating to cancer:

In 1931, a German scientist, Dr. Otto Warburg, was awarded the Nobel Prize in Medicine for proving that cancer is an anaerobic growth. The dictionary defines anaerobic as living or occurring in the absence of free oxygen. About three years later, he discovered that oxygen provided the answer to successful treatment of cancer.

WOW! Can you imagine that; a possible cure for cancer that has been around for over 75 years and almost no one knows about it? You don't suppose for a minute that THEY would suppress this valuable information for their financial gain, do you? Well, probably not unless there was a big pile of money at stake. On the other hand, the drug companies rake in almost $300 billion annually. That is a big pile of dough. In 10 years, that would amount to about $3 trillion. That kind of money could pay off the national debt in short order.

Now for more about cancer. Just because you breathe in oxygen with every breath, that does not mean that it gets down to the cellular level. Each and every cell must have oxygen to function. Every cell requires calcium and other minerals to function and to pull in the oxygen.

Linus Pauling said that EVERY ILLNESS is associated with MINERAL DEFICIENCY.

Most, if not all, cancer gets its start and growth in an organ of the body where oxygen is minimal or entirely absent. It occurs in sick, dying, damaged or dormant body tissue and organs. That explains why cancer occurs in the male prostate gland (dormant tissue), women's breasts (dormant tissue) and sunburned skin (damaged tissue).

It takes a combination of many things for cancer to occur; an accumulation of toxins (which is the main cause), the absence of oxygen, and a deficiency of minerals primarily calcium. We really need the benefit of calcium, but all the calcium in the world won't help you without magnesium and vitamin D-3. In addition, the cancer patient will always have a low pH which is very acidic (below 7.0).

If you were to ask the average person what causes cancer, you would no doubt get an answer something like this: "I don't know." I have done that with many people and that's the answer I get every time. However, everyone knows, or should know, what causes cancer. It is in the newspaper almost everyday. The answer is toxins cause cancer. How do I know? They even have a word for it. The word is carcinogen. Carcinogen means a toxin that has been known to cause cancer. Not only do we know that carcinogens cause cancer, but we know that all carcinogens are toxins. It is my theory that any toxin could be a carcinogen. To further support this idea, we also know that there has been an increase of cancer by leaps and bounds in the last 100 years. Coincidental to that increase in cancer, we also know that we have had an increase in the toxic pollution of our environment in the last 100 years.

Heart problems and cancer could be virtually eliminated if we were to treat the cause directly. If we could eliminate all the toxins from our environment, we would probably be cancer free. Additionally, the body can and does fight cancer if it's given the proper nutrition and maybe a lot of oxygen. Since we as individuals cannot eliminate all toxins from our environment, we must treat ourselves individually. What can we do?

The following paragraphs contain information about POSSIBLE cancer treatments. I'm unable to guarantee that any of them will work for you, because I have not tried them. I have never had cancer. I know what has worked for me in treating my ALS, but not cancer. Based on my ALS experience and what I've read, I BELIEVE all these treatments could possibly be effective. I personally would try any of these long before I would ever try chemotherapy or radiation. No, I cannot recommend any treatment for anyone.

We know that many toxins remain in our body a long time and accumulate. So, the first thing I would do would be to detoxify the body. There are many, many ways to detoxify the body such as: Chelation, drink lots of water, colon hydrotherapy, fasting, diet and supplements. Now supplements are important and there is one that may be more important than all others—calcium; but you need magnesium and vitamin D-3 to make it work.

If you want to know more about calcium and oxygen, here is a book you may want to read: "The Calcium Factor: the Scientific Secret of Health and Youth" by Robert R. Barefoot & Carl J. Reich, MD.

Dr. Barefoot states that JAMA, "The Journal of American Medicine Association," published an article in 2002 that stated clearly that cancer could be reversed by calcium. Why doesn't your doctor know about that? Well, probably because he never read it and doctors are not trained in nutrition. Further, they don't believe in supplements.

According to Dr. Barefoot, calcium in your body will increase the oxygen at the cellular level. Also, vitamin sunshine (vitamin D) is required for calcium to be more effective. Additionally, oxygen treatments could be a great benefit too. Another great idea would be chlorine dioxide—more on that later.

Why am I so big on calcium? Because it is helping me. I have reversed all the symptoms of a terminal illness called ALS by primarily detoxification of my body. Recently I have begun to take marine coral calcium and it has helped me improve.

Well, now you have a Nobel Prize winner, "The Journal of American Medicine Association" and Dr. Barefoot, a medical scientist, all three telling us about possible CURES for cancer. Who are you going to believe, them or YOUR doctor? The only approved cancer treatments are chemotherapy, radiation and surgery.

I believe cancer is caused by toxins and, therefore, we should eliminate the toxins in our body. Treat it with calcium and oxygen. I don't know, but this would seem very reasonable to me. There are clinics in Mexico who claim to cure cancer with diet primarily. From what I've read about their procedures, they do only a little to detoxify. I met one man who had been there and done that. He had actually improved and the cancer was in remission. However, he eventually returned to his normal diet and died about two years later. Why? I believe the answer is that not enough was done to detoxify. Remember, toxins cause cancer. I think you detoxify first, and then follow a nutritious diet to help the body heal itself.

If you want to know more about detox, you may want to know more about Chelation. If so, I would recommend the following book: "Forty Something Forever, a Consumer's Guide to Chelation Therapy and other Heart-Savers" by Harold & Arline Brecher. There is more about Chelation in a later chapter.

Over the last few years, I have read over 30 books written by health care professionals, mostly medical doctors. If you have cancer and could only read one book, here is what I would recommend: "The pH Miracle—Balance Your Diet, Reclaim Your Health" by Robert O. Young, Ph.D., and Shelley Redford Young. Here is just one example from this book: To cleanse your body *"I recommend you take several things. The two most crucial are pH drops (chlorine dioxide or hydrogen peroxide) and concentrated green powder."* For more info on chlorine dioxide, see below.

Obviously, correcting your pH to be more alkaline is critical to improving your health. Frankly, I'm not sure which comes first; sickness or acidic pH. Either way, if you take steps to improve your health, your pH will become alkaline. If you take steps to make your pH more alkaline, you will be more healthy. At any rate, you now know that cancer cannot survive in an oxygen-filled environment and it cannot survive in an alkaline environment. Acidic people have poor oxygen utilization. There will be more in later chapters about pH.

Chlorine Dioxide

According to what I have read, chlorine dioxide will seek and destroy pesticides, pathogens and EVEN CANCER cells. It will even raise your pH and help detoxify heavy metals and other toxins. Chlorine dioxide is approved by the Environmental Protection Agency for safely removing pathogens and contaminates like anthrax. It is slowly replacing chlorine for municipal water treatment systems.

THE AMERICAN SOCIETY OF ANALYTICAL CHEMISTS PROCLAIMED IN 1999 THAT CHLORINE DIOXIDE IS THE MOST POWERFUL PATHOGEN KILLER KNOWN TO MAN.

Normal levels of oxygen in the blood cannot destroy all of the pathogens, but chlorine dioxide is one part chlorine and two parts oxygen.

I could stop there, but you may be interested in knowing that there are many other cancer treatments that I have learned about. I am not a laboratory medical scientist so I am unable to tell you that these will cure cancer; BUT many medical scientists believe they can. Here they are:

Dr. Lorraine Day was for 15 years on the faculty of the University of California, San Francisco, School of Medicine as Associate Professor and Vice Chairman of the Department of Orthopedics. When she developed cancer, she had a large malignant tumor removed surgically but she refused chemotherapy and successfully treated her condition with alternative treatments. Now don't miss this folks, here is a medical doctor who refused chemotherapy and lived. Just one of her many video tapes that I recommend is "Cancer Doesn't Scare Me Anymore." To order, call toll-free 1-800-574-2437.

From what I've read, chemo kills as many as it saves. It is my personal choice to NEVER DO CHEMOTHERAPY. Even if it cures your cancer, it may have damaged many of your organs and you will probably have health problems the rest of your life.

I should mention that the same thing is true for radiation. I only know the results of one person who had cancer and was treated with radiation. Within a short two months after radiation, she had to have over $10,000 worth of dental work done; all caused by the radiation treatment. And that was only the beginning.

There are many possible cures for cancer which have been forced underground and criticized by the powers that be (and you know who). Most of them involve diet and I believe they work.

Hippocrates is well-known as the "Father of Medicine." He said *"Let food be your medicine and medicine be your food."* The following is information that I have run across about food diets that may possibly be successful in treating cancer:

The GRAPE DIET has been used for over 400 years to treat many illnesses according to a book I read. The author also claims that The Grape Diet has been known to successfully treat cancer. You can order a book titled "The Grape Cure" by Johanna Brandt from The American School of Naturopathy, Home Study Department, P.O. Box 404/Murray Hill, New York, NY 10156.

I have read that around the 1930's, they were curing cancer in the Mayo Clinic with a diet of only milk. HOWEVER, it was RAW milk straight from the cow; not pasteurized or homogenized and purely organic.

I've also read that a diet of raw organic eggs may also cure cancer.

As I mentioned earlier, increased oxygen may destroy cancer cells. However, the oxygen must reach the cellular level and the cells must be able to draw in the oxygen from your bloodstream. There are many ways to increase oxygen. One is hyperbaric oxygen treatments. Another one is ozone. Ozone is another form of oxygen (O3). This oxygen (O3) will attach to bacteria, fungi, mold, parasites and TUMORS. During this process, it oxidizes or destroys them. This oxygen has a high pH (between 7.0 and 9.0).

There is a book "Self-Treatment for AIDS, Oxygen Therapies, Etc." edited by Betsy Russell-Manning, Soft cover, 1989, ISBN #09301618. This book contains many claims by doctors in other countries who have used ozone and peroxide treatments to cure many illnesses including AIDS and cancer.

Here is still another book about a possible cancer cure: "The Gerson Therapy" by Charlotte Gerson and Morton Walker, D.P.M. The book is all about Charlotte Gerson's father, Max Gerson. In 1945, Max Gerson appeared before Congress with five people who he claimed had been cured of cancer with his treatment. I believe that there are many cancer clinics throughout the world that may be using his theories in treating cancer with fresh, raw vegetables and vegetable juices.

The Issels Treatment Center—"Complete long term remissions of advanced cancers." This is a statement found on their Internet web site:
www.issels.com/clinics/itc/

This clinic is in San Diego, California and has been there since 1951. According to their web site, they use a combination of conventional and alternative treatments. The web site includes several testimonials.

There is one more book that I would really check out if I had cancer: "How to Fight Cancer & Win" by William L. Fischer. You can order it on the web site:
www.agorahealthbooks.com

Even if you don't have cancer, you may want to visit this web site for more information about the suppression of natural cures.

DON'T MISS THIS—THIS IS REALLY BIG. (I don't know if the statements are correct, but they are what I have read more than once and I believe they are true.)

CANCER CANNOT SURVIVE IN AN OXYGEN-RICH ENVIRONMENT.

CANCER CANNOT SURVIVE IN AN ALKALINE pH ENVIRONMENT.

Assuming the above is correct, you may want to correct your pH to alkaline as well as add calcium, magnesium, and vitamin D-3. This can be done by following a more alkaline diet of fresh organic vegetables, fruits and nuts; much of it raw. Also, chlorine dioxide and/or oxygen should improve your pH.

Here are some web sites with much more information about successfully treating cancer:
http://cancerbreakthroughusa.com/order.html
hhttp://www.ozoneuniversity.com/healingowersofoxygen.htm
http://www.beating-cancer-gently.com/nl119.html

Here is one more possible cure for cancer. I have read that vitamin C in large doses can destroy cancer. Evidently you cannot take a large enough dose orally, so it must be done by IV. According to what I've read, one hospital has had success by combining vitamin C by IV along with conventional cancer treatments.

Cancer Test

Biopsies are dangerous because they can spread the cancer. Here is one way to avoid having to do a biopsy. Your doctor may never tell you, but there has been a medical test for cancer that is 99% effective that has been available for 25 years. It is more effective, less dangerous and cheaper than all other medical cancer tests. It's called AMAS cancer test. You don't have to go to a doctor; the test is available on the Internet. The cost is $165. The kit is free, you take a smear of your own blood and send it in and pay when the results are ready. The test is for specific cancer antibodies that will be present. Go to

www.oncolabinc.com.

One More Possible Cancer Cure

I've already told you about several possible cures for cancer and now I have one more. Some of these ideas for cancer treatments have been around for nearly a hundred years. This one was discovered in 1868, 140 years ago. Peter Busch, a medical doctor, discovered that cancer cannot tolerate a fever or high temperatures. And now, folks, that's what they're doing in Germany today. They claim to be curing cancer by cooking the tumor to death. They also are using not one but several types of treatments in their cancer treatment.

All this comes from a book written by Andrew Scholberg—Title "German Cancer Breakthrough."

If you have cancer or are concerned about cancer, you may want to order this book.

You may want to visit the following web site for much more information:

http://www.germancancerbreakthrough.com/B/

The author states that he has toured 17 cancer clinics in four different countries. He recommends six of them which are all in Germany. The author claims to have visited these clinics in Germany and has interviewed the doctors. He describes the many treatments they use and many of them are exactly what we have already discussed such as hypothermia, ozone, an alkaline diet, and bathing and drinking natural mineral water. I really think that it is most interesting that they are doing all the treatments that our doctors totally ignore. The book provides all the details about the six outstanding clinics and will provide you with all the phone numbers, web sites, and e-mail addresses.

Now I have no way of knowing whether or not these German doctors can cure cancer. However, all that they do sounds very logical to me. I know that my ALS condition was caused by toxins and we know that cancer is caused by toxins also. Apparently the German doctors know this too and that's why they include one or more types of treatments for detoxification. That's basically what I did to keep myself alive. To the best of my knowledge, most American doctors never do this and that's why many cancer patients have a reoccurrence of their cancer. Again, we should logically do something to treat the cause.

The author also claims that many celebrities from the U.S. have been treated and cured for cancer in Germany. These celebrities include former President Ronald Reagan who went to Dr. Hans Nieper in Germany in May of 1985.

Let's review this and give it a little more thought. You can't help but wonder if these cancer clinics in Germany really do cure anyone. I have given that a lot of thought and I believe they do primarily because what they do is very logical. One example is that among their many treatments is one that was discovered by an American doctor over 100 years ago. Further, here is a list of things that they do differently than our doctors do here in America: Detoxification, you drink and bathe in mineral water, nutritious diet and if they ever use chemo, it's a very low dose. They also rarely do any surgery.

Their treatments are all LOGICAL and correspond to the many things that I have done to treat my so-called terminal illness. Remember, more than one medical doctor told me that my ALS was incurable and I proved them all wrong. Most of our doctors here in the U.S. know nothing about toxins or how to eliminate toxins. Toxins are the primary cause of ALS and cancer so the treatments do correspond.

Make note that there is not one but six clinics providing similar treatments for cancer.

They not only provide treatments which may cure, but also they treat the cause. Most American doctors do not do that. That's why many cancer patients in America have cancer reoccurrences.

One of the best things is that none of their treatments cause any harm. The German doctors must be practicing the Hippocratic Oath and most American doctors violate that oath everyday.

Their treatments cost in the area of 10% of what cancer treatments cost here in the U.S.

Here in America, we have been treating cancer basically the same way for well over 50 years. Years ago, my boss had a quote hanging on his office wall that went something like this: "If you have been doing something the same way for 15 or 20 years, there is good reason to think that there must be a better way."

Another really important thing about the German clinic is that nothing they do is painful or damaging to the patient. On the other hand, EVERYTHING we do to treat cancer is damaging and life threatening and that includes surgery, radiation and chemo. All three treatments violate the Hippocratic Oath.

All this information convinces me that we may be avoiding cancer treatments that could cure.

Do you think this information indicates corruption in our medical system?

If I had cancer today or if I wanted to PREVENT cancer, I would try correcting my pH to alkaline and taking chlorine dioxide and other detox treatments including colon hydrotherapy. I believe that would do it, but if it did not, I would be on a plane to Germany.

Another good idea to prevent cancer is to be sure that you are getting enough vitamin C in your diet. Here is a good way to add some vitamin C to your daily diet: Make a drink with the juice of one lemon, add a little maple syrup (not artificial) or honey, and add about 12 oz. of pure water and a pinch of cayenne pepper.

I just read a book titled "The Cure" by Dr. Timothy Brantley. Now don't miss this. Here is a doctor who writes about treating one of his first cancer patients by diet, herbs and correcting the pH. The patient's tumor completely disappeared and that story would tend to confirm some of the previous stories in this chapter.

Resveratrol

I have read a report written by a medical doctor which said that Resveratrol can inhibit the growth of cancer cells and even kill them.

Asparagus and Cancer

It may be hard to believe but another possible cancer treatment has recently come to my attention. An article entitled "Asparagus for cancer" allegedly was printed in "The Cancer News Journal" in December 1979. The article included several case studies of successful treatment of cancer with asparagus. Now I have no idea whether or not this is true, but it sounds very interesting to me and also quite possibly true. I won't go into all the stories, but they are quite convincing.

Here is the treatment:

The asparagus must be cooked and then placed in a blender and liquefied to make a puree. Take four full tablespoons of the puree twice daily. You may take it hot or cold and diluted or not.

I know from personal experience that asparagus is truly a unique food. It is the ONLY food that will change the odor of your urine and it will do that in a very short time after you eat it. This indicates to me that asparagus may have unique healing properties.

You might be laughing at the idea that asparagus can cure cancer, but I would not rely on it entirely. There are too many other elements that effect cancer such as toxins. Additionally, here are some facts about asparagus: Asparagus contains a good supply of protein called histones, which are believed to be active in controlling cell growth. Asparagus is said to contain a substance that we will call cell growth normalizer. Asparagus is the highest tested food containing glutathione, which is one of the body's most potent ANTICARCINOGENS and ANTIOXIDANTS.

Conclusion

This chapter has suggested how to avoid cancer, how to possibly cure cancer and how to test for cancer, all by yourself. All you must do is believe it's possible.

ALL THESE POTENTIAL CURES FOR CANCER LEAD ME TO BELIEVE THAT AT LEAST ONE OR MORE MAY WORK. I DON'T BELIEVE THAT ANY ILLNESS IS INCURABLE. THAT'S NOT LOGICAL.

Now here is a major point and don't miss this: Although there is no hard evidence that any of these cancer treatments will actually cure, there is also no hard evidence THAT THEY WON'T CURE. There are no provisions in our entire medical system to prove or disprove any NATURAL treatment.

If you love your MD and/or believe our medical system cannot be wrong, then you may be questioning all the above possible cancer cures. You may even think that they are all hocus-pocus dominocus and totally nuts. You may even think I am nuts. However, if I'm nuts, then I am in good company. Remember that it was the father of medicine, Hippocrates, who said that *"Food is medicine."* Also, most of the books listed in Chapter 4 were written by MD's and most of those MD's would agree with me. Now for the clincher: In Chapter 5, I mention that Dr. Ignarro was awarded a Nobel Prize in Medicine for his discovery on the benefits of Nitric Oxide. Now guess what makes your body produce more Nitric Oxide: Certain FOODS.

If you are still scratching your head in wonderment, and you think that if this was all true then most of our MD's would know about it. Well, all I can say is this:

ALMOST ALL MEDICAL DOCTORS HAVE A STRONG PREFERENCE FOR PRESCRIPTION DRUGS AND THEY REFUSE TO EVEN LOOK AT OR CONSIDER ANY ALTERNATIVE TREATMENT. That would be OK except for the fact that MOST DRUGS DO NOT CURE. Therefore, the only place you can look for any possible cure is alternative treatments other than drugs.

You may be having a lot of trouble accepting this new idea, so let me explain what has happened. It is my belief that the drug companies have been brain washing the doctors and the public that their way is the only way and you and I are simply victims of the brain washing.

Here is one more thought. All the evidence has convinced me that there is a law that prevents anyone from COMMUNICATING that their treatment or pill can actually CURE cancer or any illness. In other words, even if I knew and could confirm that one of these treatments could actually cure cancer, I would not dare tell you in this book. It is literally against the law to use the word "cure" or the "Medical Mafia" will descend upon you like locusts on a wheat field. In a democracy, no one should fear the government. Well, I fear the government in this situation. Every time I use the words "possible cure," I cringe a little. Glenna and I are both deadly afraid of what may happen to us when this book is published.

Health care in the U.S.A. is all about money and not about cures. Just because most doctors don't believe there are cancer cures, DOES THAT MEAN THAT NO CURES EXIST?

CHAPTER 7

PRESCRIPTION DRUGS

I wonder how many people realize that prescription drugs DO NOT provide a cure (with rare exceptions)?

Welcome to the HEART of this book.

To begin with, it is simply not logical to treat ALL ILLNESS with drugs and yet that's what we are doing. Using a drug for most health problems is just like putting a band-aid on a leak in your water pipe. The band-aid might slow the leak and hide it, but it will not fix it or cure it. Is that what you really intend to do?

To the best of my knowledge, all prescription drugs are TOXIC. Toxin is just another word meaning poison. It is not logical to take a poison for a long period of time and expect your health to improve.

In a recent article about an interview with an old man, age 107, the writer asked this obvious question: *"To what do you attribute your longevity?"*

The 107 year old man said *"I believe you must remain ACTIVE and stay away from PRESCRIPTION DRUGS."*

I'm not 107, but I could not agree more.

Before I tear into the drug problem, I want to remind you that there are some good prescription drugs.

Drugs which are used during surgery are of vital importance to us and they are absolutely necessary. There are other drugs which may be used in life threatening situations which are also vitally important. Also, there are a few drugs, but only a few, which may be taken long-term and which may benefit the patient.

Let's look now at the benefits of a few drugs. You will often hear the drug companies make this statement in their TV commercials: *"The benefits are worth the risk."* Generally, I believe that's not true. One reason I say that is because they don't tell you what the risk is. In my opinion, they downplay the real risk. Nonetheless, there are SOME drugs which are truly worth the risk.

When I was a kid and first developed asthma, they had no drug or treatment. I would just stay up all night in a sitting position working as hard as I could to continue breathing and stay alive. I could not breathe lying down. Later, they developed a little green pill that works wonders. After taking only one pill, my breathing would return to normal within a few minutes. To me, that was a wonder drug.

I've had an off and on back problem for years and years. One time Glenna and I and our daughter Raylene were headed for a one week vacation in Baja Mexico. We left Friday night and stopped north of the border for a nights sleep. In the morning, I went for a walk to stretch my legs when suddenly I was stricken with severe and I mean severe back pain. I struggled back into the camper and Glenna began driving us home, because there was no way I would continue on our vacation with my back pain. Glenna gave me two Codeine and Tylenol pills and I lay down while she began driving home. After thirty minutes, I told her to turn around. I felt so good from the Codeine/Tylenol that I was certain I would be OK on our vacation and I was! Conclusion: I love Codeine/Tylenol.

OK, there are two stories about two drugs that are better than just GOOD.

Here is a third story that will prove that the benefits outweigh the risk SOMETIMES. Glenna's mother was 90 years old about two years ago and had a stroke. She was completely paralyzed on the right side. Glenna found her in her chair leaning over to the right, drooling from the mouth, and unable to speak. She was rushed to the hospital. The diagnosis was grim. There was only one hope and that was a drug called a "clot buster." The benefit of the drug is that it would dissolve the blood clot and prevent further brain damage. The risk is possible death. The doctor said he had never prescribed that drug for anyone her age, but his best estimate was that there was a 15% chance of death within the hour if she took the drug. If not, she would probably remain paralyzed the rest of her life. The family decided that Thelma would not want to live like that and they all agreed to try the drug, and they did. Thelma did not die and she had a miraculous recovery that began within minutes. That folks is a true example of *"the benefits are worth the risk."*

Now, we probably all agree that there are some good drugs but I believe the only good ones are ones that we take short term as in all three stories. However, I am totally convinced that taking any one of most of the drugs on the market for a long period of time is wrong. The reason I believe that is because there are other ways to treat illness other than prescription drugs. Also, and more than that, drugs do not cure (with few exceptions like antibiotics). I like the ring of that so let me repeat it.

MOST DRUGS DON'T CURE.

Most people are probably not aware of that, AND the doctors will rarely tell you that. I never had a doctor tell me that. Most drugs have only a TEMPORARY effect.

Here is one more thing about prescription drugs and the reason why they don't cure. Except for the antibiotics, most drugs do not treat the CAUSE. I like the ring of that also, so I will repeat it.

MOST DRUGS DO NOT TREAT THE CAUSE OF ILLNESS.

Let's use aspirin as an example although aspirin no longer requires a prescription. It is still a legal drug. Probably everyone gets a headache occasionally and takes an aspirin for it. I have no problem with that, but only if it's occasional. If you have headaches frequently, then you must understand that aspirin DOES NOT treat the CAUSE of the headache. Frequent headaches may indicate a serious health problem. Continued use of this drug may result in more severe health problems. Long term use of aspirin kills almost 2,000 people every year in the U.S.

Here is one more fact about prescription drugs that many people do not realize. Drugs are dangerous. Oh I like that one too. Let me repeat it.

ALL PRESCRIPTION DRUGS ARE DANGEROUS.

If they were still alive, there are many celebrities who could vouch for that; including Elvis Presley, Anna Nicole Smith and Heath Ledger.

And now folks we have another one in late June 2009. Michael Jackson has died at the age of 50 from cardiac arrest. From several live interviews on TV, it is my conclusion that Michael may have died from one or more prescription drugs. They may blame it on a "overdose" and that may or may not be correct. Evidently he has been taking several prescription drugs for a long time. I think sometimes our medical doctors truly forget just how dangerous these drugs are when taken long term.

Why do most drugs require a prescription? Answer: Because of the fact that they are dangerous. Well, you may be thinking this:

"Eric, I've been taking drugs all my life and no problem yet." My answer is that you are one of the lucky ones. Just wait, time will tell.

Let's look first at what they say in one of their TV commercials. There is a drug used for erectile dysfunction (E. D.). They warn you about taking other drugs or drinking alcohol at the same time. I have to laugh at this part. They also tell you to call your doctor if your erection lasts longer than four hours. What in the world do you do with one that lasts one, two or three hours? I can't imagine.

Here is the part that really gets me. They say that continued use of that drug may cause headaches, upset stomach, and delayed backache (I don't know what they mean by delayed). Then they go on to say call your doctor if any sudden loss of hearing or vision. Wow, now get this. Here is a drug that is totally UNNECESSARY. You are not in a life threatening situation. In fact, I would classify this as a RECREATIONAL drug.

According to what I've read, these E. D. drugs are only effective on half of the men taking them. That doesn't sound too good to me, considering the cost and the intolerable side effects to the men.

Let me repeat one of their warnings in my interpretation using my own words.

Call your doctor if you begin TO GO BLIND OR LOSE YOUR HEARING. *"Wait a minute, Eric, did they really say that?"* Well, they said loss of vision and I interpret that as going blind. Here is my point to all this. I think people trust their doctors not to give them anything that is dangerous and further most people completely ignore the warnings. They believe what the drug companies frequently say *"The risk is worth the benefit."* In this case, I do not think that's true. Again, we have a totally unnecessary drug that may cause you to go blind. Is that risk really worth the benefit? I don't think so.

This is just one example of a dangerous drug if taken long term.

When the drug companies warn you of all this, they are doing it for their own benefit. If someone or their product causes you injury, you may file a lawsuit against them for damages. However, if they warned you ahead of time, then you may have no case. If they FAILED TO WARN you, then you may have a case.

Did you ever hear of Murphy's Law? *"Whatever can go wrong, will go wrong."* I believe that Murphy's Law may apply to prescription drugs. They always say something like these possible side effects are rare. However, they only test their drugs for a relatively short length of time. They have no idea what the long-term effects may be. I believe there is a high probability that Murphy's Law will prove to be correct, and that sooner or later you will have these side effects.

In all of their warnings, I rarely hear them admit that their drug may be fatal. However, they are admitting that more and more lately. My ALS condition was caused by a prescription drug and ALS is 99% of the time fatal. No one ever told me that the drug Flagyl could kill me. I never heard that, but it almost did.

Some of the drug commercials on TV have lengthy warnings about the serious side effects. All you have to do is listen carefully and you will realize just how dangerous they are. Is anyone listening?

Now, for a few statistics that may blow your mind. I've never seen all of these figures in one article, but they have appeared in newspaper articles individually:

About 90,000 people die annually from errors in filling the prescription order.

Approximately 110,000 die every year from one or more drugs administered in the hospital. These figures are based on VOLUNTARY reporting.

Now, that's a total of about 200,000 deaths a year from drugs. Does that prove to you that drugs are dangerous? Maybe it does, but wait a minute, that's not all. These are voluntary reports and knowing human nature, there must be many more which are not reported. There could easily be double this amount. Also, these are only deaths which occur IN THE HOSPITAL. How many occur outside the hospital? We simply don't know. I think these deaths in the hospital are usually from one drug only, but how many occur from taking multiple drugs away from the hospital? That could be an enormous figure.

The drug used for chemotherapy is highly toxic and if you survive it, you may have many health problems in the future. According to an article I read written by a medical doctor, he said that around half of the chemo treated patients will die from the chemotherapy. I have not read any actual figures, but that must be in the area of another 100,000 a year or more.

Here is one more situation we must add to this equation:

Let's take all the warnings on any one drug and multiply that by 10 or 12. Most people are taking 10 or more drugs daily in the U.S. In addition to that, pour in the possibility of interaction between two or more drugs. When you begin interpolating the known figures, you may have a very, very large figure. To my way of thinking, the total number of deaths in the U.S. could very well be in the area of 500,000 to ONE MILLION every year. Did you know that one and a half million people are hospitalized every year from prescription drugs? There is no doubt many more people suffer serious side effects and are not hospitalized.

The obituaries interest me and I read them now and then just to know the age and cause of death. I read them often and have done that for many years. Neither Glenna nor I have ever seen the cause of death to be PRESCRIPTION DRUGS.

Add to all the above this fact: This is a quote from an article in the "Los Angeles Times" on 10-23-08:

"*The number of deaths and serious injury associated with prescription drug use rose to record levels in the first quarter of this year.*" The article went on to say the number of deaths and serious injuries rose 38% from last year's quarterly average. The article also said that the most dangerous drug was the anti-smoking drug Varenicline. Now, how irrational and illogical is that? You are taking a drug to avoid dying from smoking and yet the drug may kill you. In my book, you might as well keep smoking and enjoy it. What the hell is the difference? Just so you know, heparin, a blood thinner, was the second most deadly drug. I would avoid that like the Black Plague.

It is simply not logical that only a drug can treat illness. It is not logical that there are not at least SOME NATURAL treatments. For the most part, medical doctors in the U.S.A. exclusively prescribe drugs in treating illness.

Let me give you just one example of natural treatments. First of all, I believe it is always best to know and treat the CAUSE of any problem rather than some other idea. If I remember correctly back when I was just a kid, they called it SUGAR DIABETES. Now that indicates to me that sugar must have something to do with diabetes. For obvious reasons, they have dropped the word "sugar." At any rate, diabetes is probably caused by a poor diet, too much sugar and maybe triggered by an overload of toxic heavy metals. Wouldn't it make more sense to treat the cause of the problem rather than taking a drug?

One of the problems is that you cannot obtain a patent on a natural substance like a vitamin or mineral. Additionally, the FDA only approves substances that can be patented.

Many drugs, long before they were approved as a drug, were developed from NATURAL CURES. For example, the bark of a tree was made into a powder and was taken internally to reduce pain from headaches. Later, the drug companies developed a similar synthetic product that became known as aspirin. Aspirin, like most drugs, can be fatal. Did you know that aspirin is responsible for almost 2,000 deaths a year in the U.S.?

In all probability Michael Jackson was addicted to sedatives and painkillers and that may have been responsible for his death. No doubt there are many more of us who are addicted to prescription drugs. I read recently that the number of prescriptions for painkiller drugs increased from 40 million to 180 million in just 15 years. That amazes me because that's over 400%. Also the number of prescriptions for sleeping pills went up 54% in the last four years. I really hope those people know that they are making "mucho" money for the drug companies and in the long run they will be the losers.

My one major conclusion about drugs is that taking multiple drugs over a long period of time is a death sentence. You probably will never get well.

This entire chapter can be summed up with this. The overuse of prescription drugs is the direct cause of three things:

1. An enormous number of deaths measured in six figures every year.
2. An enormous number of people with chronic illness that drugs cannot cure.
3. The overall costs of medical treatment is so large that it has a major negative effect on our entire economy.

Thinking only of the economy, I pray *"Oh God, please don't let them expand medical insurance to cover more people before we make major repairs to our busted medical care system."*

Remember, this was all predicted over 200 years ago and it was predicted by a medical doctor.

At the beginning of this chapter, I told you about the 107 year old man. Since I wrote this chapter, it has occurred to me that my family has a history of longevity, nearly as old, AND ALL WITHOUT ANY PRESCRIPTION DRUGS.

My maternal great grandmother died at age 99.

Both grandmothers lived into their late 90's.

My uncle Cyril lived to be 92.

My aunt Meda really takes the cake and I know more about her. She not only lived to be 98, but she lived her entire life without ever seeing a medical doctor and without ever taking ANY drug, not even an aspirin.

Also, she never had a sick day in her life and never was a patient in a hospital other than childbirth.

It is a common thought that we are living longer than previous generations. I believe it may be statistically correct but only because of antibiotics which were developed in the first half of the 20th century. I don't believe that we have made any progress since then.

The drug companies often say in their TV commercials that the drug side effects are RARE. I wonder how they define rare. We think they are minimizing that problem unrealistically. We believe that serious side effects occur much more often than they imply by the use of the word RARE.

Taking a prescription drug for an illness is just exactly the same as taking a pain pill for a broken leg. The pain pill does not cure the broken leg, but it does make you feel better.

WAKE UP AMERICA… Consider alternative treatments.

Taking prescription drugs, in my opinion, is only one step better than taking rat poison. By the way, rat poison will cure any illness and it's far less expensive; what I mean is death cures all.

Although the use of prescription drugs in our country is excessive, there are benefits from carefully prescribed and monitored prescription drugs, but only when used judiciously and for a LIMITED time period.

CHAPTER 8

THE DRUG COMPANIES—BIG PHARMA

(I could have called them the pharmaceutical corporations, but that's too classy)

"Boston Legal" was one of our favorite TV shows. It was not only entertaining, but informative about newsworthy items such as gun control, gay marriage, etc. Another reason I liked their shows is because I generally agree with their point of view. Not long ago they had a program all about the tobacco industry and one week later they had another show about the pharmaceutical companies. It is my purpose to let you know what they said about Big Tobacco and about Big Pharma before I say anything more.

Let's start first with Big Tobacco, so you can get an idea of what any type of large corporation can and will do for money. In the beginning of the one hour "Boston Legal" TV show, there was a discussion among the attorneys about why even take a case against a tobacco company. They said no one ever really wins and a law firm could go bankrupt before they would ever have their day in court. The tobacco company will always play the DELAY GAME and drag it out for years and years. They also discussed that the tobacco industry was systematically killing people. During the trial, one witness blamed her dad's death on smoking. The plaintiff's attorneys said that CIGARETTES KILL ONE-THIRD TO ONE-HALF OF THEIR CUSTOMERS; one death every six seconds.

Here are more statements made during the two TV shows:

They said the tobacco companies and the pharmaceutical companies were very similar.

They both deny their products harm people.

They both promote INDEPENDENT research that they pay for (if Big Pharma pays for the research, how can you call it independent?)

They both spend millions on lobbyists.

They both suppress information that their products kill people.

They pointed out that there is one difference. The FDA is hostile to Big Tobacco, but they roll over for Big Pharma.

Big Pharma has been caught bribing.

Big Pharma spends twice as much on promotion than they spend on research and development.

The TV audience is exposed to 16 hours a year of TV commercials about drug products.

They accused Big Pharma of inventing diseases for which they can provide a drug treatment.

Further, they said Big Pharma is totally out of control and the FDA turns their back on it.

This is the end of the comments from the first two "Boston Legal" TV shows. A few weeks later, they had another show which included some hair raising remarks about Big Pharma. On 10-27-08 ABC had another show and the following comments are taken directly from that broadcast. These comments were made by the "Boston Legal" attorney to the jury:

"You know the death grip the pharmaceutical industry has on this country. They've infiltrated the FDA. Studies showed that 90% of all FDA advisory meetings had at least one person with ties to Big Pharmaceutical."

"And then there's Congress. Big Pharma have given members of Congress $70 million since 1990."

"A famed Harvard psychiatrist helped fuel the recent boom in anti-psychotics (drugs) for kids. Turns out he personally took over $1.6 million from drug makers over the past seven years. He also failed to report this income to the university."

THAT'S REALLY DISTURBING TO ME, and I hope that is to you too. My opinion is that is just criminal. Just think what they are doing to our kids in order for them to make a profit. There will be more about our kids later.

Shortly after these episodes on tobacco and Big Pharma, "Boston Legal" ceased to exist. I WONDER WHY?

This is the end of the material from "Boston Legal."

*   *   *

All major drug or pharmaceutical companies that I know of are corporations and most corporations exist to make a profit. The corporations are owned by the stockholders. Large corporations have hundreds or thousands of stockholders.

These stockholders are expecting the corporation to make a profit. Of even greater importance, these stockholders are anticipating more profits this year than last year. In other words, they want the company to grow its earnings so the stock value will go up and at some future date they could sell their stock at a profit. These stockholders appoint a management team to run the corporation. The stockholders provide no moral or legal guidance. They simply want the management to grow the earnings. This arrangement sometimes causes management to make decisions based on profit and not on morality or legality. In other words, large amounts of money can influence people to lie, cheat and steal.

Drug companies have a really tough row to hoe. It costs millions of dollars and takes several years to bring a single drug to market. Once they have invested all this time and money, they simply must bring it to market to hopefully get their money back plus a profit. Also, the patent is only good for a few years (usually twenty years). Due to the overall cost to develop drugs, they simply cannot compete with any natural treatment such as an inexpensive vitamin or mineral product. Evidence would indicate that they will do everything in their power to fight and DESTROY all competition. You and I know this because they have done a good job in convincing most of the world that their drugs are far superior to any NATURAL product. BUT, that cannot be true because most drugs DO NOT treat the cause.

Imagine for a moment that you are a CEO of a large pharmaceutical corporation. The head of your research department tells you that he has developed two new drugs and they are both ready for market.

Drug #1 is a treatment for cancer and it has proven to be a complete cure for cancer. The patient must take the drug everyday for 90 days for full recovery.

Drug #2 only treats the symptoms and does not cure. The patient must continue this drug the rest of his or her life.

Now think of all the ramifications to your decision. Which one will you choose?

During the last several decades, the drug companies have been the darlings of Wall Street. Why? Because of their rapid growth in earnings or profit. They can only continue their rapid growth if they sell more and more drugs to a larger and larger customer base. THEY HAVE AN INHERENT NEED FOR MORE AND MORE OF US TO GET SICK AND REMAIN SICK.

Some people want us to believe we're living longer as a result of all the "miracle drugs" we have. The only thing miracle about drugs is the fact that there are so many that don't cure. In the first half of the 20th century, our biggest health problems were infectious disease. Antibiotic drugs like penicillin have saved a lot of lives, particularly babies and young children, and that statistically increased our life expectancy. But in the last half of the 20th century, infectious diseases are no longer a MAJOR health problem. Drugs are not the answer for our other health problems and they do not contribute to our longevity; in fact, they do just the reverse. To the best of my knowledge, all the hundreds of life insurance companies are still using the 1958 Mortality Tables.

In the 1930's and 1940's, no one in my entire family took any prescription drugs. Today, the AVERAGE per person number of PRESCRIPTIONS each year is over 12. At their present rate of growth, that number could be 15 or 20 in a few short years.

A massive article on the drug companies appeared in "The Los Angeles Times" 8-6-07. In 1999, the total U.S. sales for all drug companies was $125.1 billion. In 2006, the total sales jumped to $278.8 billion. WOW! In less than 10 years, their sales more than doubled. Does that mean that we are now healthier? I don't think so. It should be noted that during that same time frame, money spent on promotions went from $13.9 billion to $27.9 billion. Note the promotion expense paralleled the increase in sales.

Big Pharma has lobbyists in Washington who outnumber Senators five to one. Lobbyists and members of the Congress include some of the best people money can buy.

Companies that market NATURAL products to treat cancer, and other serious illnesses have little chance for long-term survival. Many have been put out of business by the FDA or FTC. Here are two just for example: Lane Labs in 2004 and a company who sold a product called Coral Calcium. To the best of my knowledge, these companies' products never harmed anyone. The only thing these two companies did wrong was becoming too successful. Some large corporations simply do not want any competition.

Malpractice insurance provides the medical doctor protection in the event he or she makes a serious mistake in treating a patient. The State Insurance Department requires evidence of paid and reserved claims before considering any increase in insurance premiums. Doctors' malpractice insurance is sky high and has now become a MAJOR operating expense for doctors. Doctors must be making a lot of mistakes, so don't blame the insurance company. Many insurance companies have backed out of malpractice insurance because it is so volatile.

Here are some basic FACTS about MONEY:

ALL publicly held corporations exist to make a profit. The day-to-day goal of the top managers is to increase their profits in order to keep their million dollar jobs. The best way to increase their profit is to sell more to their present customers AND, more importantly, increase the number of their customers. This works quite well for most products, but it FAILS MISERABLY when it comes to prescription drugs.

This profit-driven system literally FORCES all employees involved in health care to work to make more money for their employer. No one person could ever stop this juggernaut.

This system provides absolutely no motivation for developing a cure. They will make more money if they never cure anyone of anything. They have developed, and the FDA has approved, well over 10,000 prescription drugs in the last few decades. Not one of them, to my knowledge, provides a CURE. Can that be accidental? By not curing anyone, the number of sick people will increase. That means that the number of their customers will increase.

The next story about the drug companies begins with a story about nylon. Around 1940 when I was about 12 years old, they invented nylon. To my knowledge the first product made with nylon was ladies stockings. Prior to that, women wore SILK stockings. Back in those days almost all the women wore them. There was a major problem with silk stockings. If you snagged them on any rough surface, they would separate by as much as a quarter of an inch and that RUN would move all up or down the stocking from top to bottom. Well, that meant another pair of silk stockings hit the trash. That was a major expense for women in those days and remember we were still recovering from the 1929 Depression.

When the new NYLON stockings were first introduced, they sold like hot cakes. The ladies soon learned that nylon simply would never run. They wore like iron. However, that did not last long. I don't know that this really happened, but it sure appears that way to me. As a result of the long-wearing nylon, sales began to fall off once every lady had a few pairs. I think the makers of the nylon stockings realized they had shot themselves in the foot. Regardless of why, nylon stockings soon began to develop runs much more often. They were still better than silk, but not as good as they were in the beginning. Now remember this happened in the early 1940's.

About that same time, Big Pharma developed penicillin, a cure for many infectious diseases. Penicillin was hailed as a miracle drug. Then, the Salk vaccine was created and that meant the end for polio. Here is what I think happened as a result of these two drugs. By eliminating many infectious diseases and polio, the income to doctors and hospitals took a big drop. Big Pharma may have learned a lesson from the nylon story and concluded that developing a drug that would cure an illness was not in their best interest. At any rate, they have not developed a cure for any illness since then. If a cure had been developed for any significant illness, it should have made headlines and you and I would know about it. I have not heard about one, have you? Now, think about that for a minute; no new cures for over 50 years.

My prediction about the future is this: As long as we have a profit-driven medical care system, our problem will remain as it is now and there will be no NEW CURES for another 50 years. Further, if you are donating money to medical research, you better think twice before you donate more. That must be the world's worse investment, with no appreciable return or benefit.

Do you like kids? I do. I love kids. One thing really neat about kids is that they are so trusting. They trust most all adults and their lives are literally in our hands. I have a powerful belief that we as adults have a tremendous obligation to protect our children; not just yours and mine, but everyone's. Obviously the drug companies do not share my feeling about our kids. Here is why I say that.

There was a newsworthy discussion on TV recently about children's vaccinations on Fox news on 6-6-08 at 10:00 PM with Greta Van-Susteren. Greta was interviewing Jenny McCarthy whose 2 1/2 year old son was diagnosed with Autism in 2005. Yes, Jenny McCarthy has been featured in "Playboy Magazine." However, she's no bimbo. I think she's pretty bright. She believes that all the toxins which are in our vaccinations are the main cause of Autism. According to her, vaccinations have in the past contained Mercury, Aluminum, Antifreeze and ether. Also, many of these toxins are still in vaccinations and shots that we continue to give our children. We could make a strong case against these toxins ever being used in this manner in the first place. However, that's not the point. The point is they are still being used.

It is very difficult to prove what causes Autism or any illness. But, let's look at the possibilities and use just one toxin—Mercury—for example. Mercury is a neuro toxin. They call it a neuro toxin because it can cause damage to the nervous system. They call Autism a neuro illness because the nervous system has been damaged. Are you beginning to get suspicious? I hope so. My ALS condition was caused by a prescription drug which is a neuro toxin. ALS is a neuro illness. I have proven beyond any doubt in my mind that Mercury and other neuro toxins can and do cause neuro degenerative illnesses such as ALS, Autism, MS, Alzheimer's, etc.

There is clearly a strong probability that Mercury and other neuro toxins in our vaccinations are causing Autism. To my knowledge, most Autism occurs AFTER vaccinations. Knowing this is a possibility, should we not err on the side of caution? In other words, I would think that if there were any possibility that the drugs would cause Autism, that the drug companies would eliminate it. HOWEVER, THEY JUST WON'T DO IT WITHOUT A FIGHT. Their defense is always *"You can't prove it."*

Let me remind you again that our children TRUST us. We have every obligation to protect them and we're not doing it. The schools require all children to have vaccinations and shots before they can enter school. There are exceptions, but hard to come by and most people are not aware of it. As the number of vaccinations and shots has increased over the years, so has the frequency of Autism.

Do we really have to prove that a toxin is poison before the drug companies will give in?

Jenny McCarthy was bright enough to learn from the mothers of other Autistic children and follow their lead. She treated her son with a gluten-free diet, by detoxifying the body and avoiding toxins. Coincidentally, that's exactly what I did to successfully treat my ALS condition. Jenny also claims that thousands of mothers have done the same thing. When are we going to wake up to the fact that Autism could very well be caused by these vaccinations? I might add that none of us are opposed to the vaccinations. We are only opposed to the toxic heavy metals like Mercury which are in them.

Here is more information from the interview that may help you. In 1983 they had a 10 shot schedule and now in 2008 it is up to 36 shots. Is that a money maker or what? Could it be that they are overdoing it just a bit?

You may demand your own shot schedule, and definitely not 10 or more at one time. Jenny recommends one shot at a time.

You can demand shots that contain no Mercury

OK, so much for vaccinations. Now, let's talk about prescribing drugs for our kids. Here is what's happening. A mother takes her bratty little kid to the doctor and complains that he is hyperactive. The doctor says *"Well, we have a solution for that—DRUG HIM."* I think that's CRIMINAL, except for extreme, extreme cases. I am violently opposed to prescription drugs for long-term treatment for adults. But, it makes me a raving lunatic to think that we are DRUGGING OUR CHILDREN. I simply can't believe the logic. Since when has the medical doctor become an expert on how to raise your and my children? From what I've read, children do not like the drugs and many of them quit taking them after a while. I don't blame them. It's not normal. It will never cure them.

Can you recall how many young children have taken their guns to school and shot and killed a number of people? This was unheard of when I was a kid; virtually non-existent. There is a strange coincidence in drugging our children and the shooting incidents. I read an article that explains one possibility. In almost every incident, the kids doing the shooting had previously been on prescription drugs and had recently quit taking them. This also is coincidental with many teenage suicides. Do you see where I'm going with this? I think we should make it a criminal offense to prescribe drugs for children, other than situations involving physical health problems. How can they possibly grow up and be physically and mentally normal if they are drugged all the time? Perhaps for the exceptional cases we should include in the law a provision for the use of a drug with court approval. In other words, you must prove to the court that the drug is necessary.

I have talked about psychiatric drugs and their effect on our children, but if you want to learn more about these drugs and their effect on adults and children, then you should visit this web site:

http://breggin.com/index.php?option=com_frontpage&Itemid=1

If you visit the above web site, you will find a lot of information about a Peter R. Breggin, MD. He has been called "the conscience of psychiatry." He is a Harvard-trained psychiatrist and has a private practice in Ithaca, New York. He has authored many articles and books. The title of some of his books will give you an idea of what he thinks about our current treatment of mental health problems:

"Medication Madness"

"Brain-Disabling Treatments in Psychiatry"

"Toxic Psychiatry"

Do the titles of those three books tell you anything?

Here is a story that just frosts my pumpkin! I don't want to mess it up, so I will quote exactly what Dr. David Williams said in his monthly newsletter "Alternatives" in October 2008: *In what has to be one of the stupidest suggestions I've ever seen, the American Academy of Pediatrics has recommended that children at age 2 have cholesterol levels tested. And then, if they have a family history of cardiovascular disease (it's the leading killer in this country—who doesn't have someone in their family with the problem?) and their cholesterol isn't "normal" they should be started on statin drugs as young as eight years old. Unbelievable.* All I can say is NOT MY KIDS.

Yes, I agree, TOTALLY UNBELIEVABLE. Just how influential are the drug companies?

Never underestimate the power of money.

All right, that's all for the kids. Now let's talk about the drug companies and their so-called clinical studies. Here are the results of a study of flu vaccinations: One group received flu vaccinations and another group (equal number) did not. Only 8% of the flu vaccination group died and 15% of the other group died. At first blush, you would conclude that the flu vaccines were effective. However, a closer look clearly indicated that the group receiving the vaccination were a much healthier group than those not receiving it.

Now here is a real eye-opener. If you are paying for the study and you want a certain outcome, you can manipulate the study anyway you want to get the results you want. You can do this a number of ways. You can select a healthier group for your drug test and an unhealthy bunch for the control group. I have heard that when one member of the study group develops a health problem, you can have him drop out and that will not affect the study. You can also provide one group with a healthier diet than the other for just one example. Again, anyway you slice it, if you are paying for and controlling the study, you can control the results to be whatever you want.

There is one more thing that the drug companies can do to muddy the waters about the efficacy of any drug. Here is an exact quote from an article in the "Los Angeles Times" which was based on a report in the "New England Journal of Medicine:"

"Nearly one-third of anti-depressant drug studies are never published in the medical literature, and nearly all happen to show that the drug being tested did not work."

Whoa there cowboy! Did that say what I think it said? I'm still catching my breath. That is quite a statement and accusation. In other words, if the study of their drug does not come out to their satisfaction, they just throw it away and do a new study. Wow! Isn't that unethical?

While we're talking about anti-depressant drugs, there is a TV drug commercial that says about two-thirds of those being treated for depression are still depressed. Well, that doesn't sound too good for the anti-depressant drugs, does it? You know, watching TV drug commercials make me want to throw up. This one I'm talking about really makes me sick when I listen to all the potential side effects. I can't imagine why anyone in their right mind would take that drug after hearing all the reasons why they should not take it. If I recall correctly, they state twice that one of the possible side effects may be DEATH. Well, that would certainly cure your depression, wouldn't it?

Here are three items which may explain the lack of integrity with our present profit-driven medical care system. They are Monopoly, The Law, and Killing Competition. Let's discuss each one.

Monopoly

Monopolies usually DO NOT work in favor of the consumer.

They almost always work to the benefit of the controlling interest in the monopoly.

The FDA and the medical doctors have monopolistic control over all INSURED medical treatment. Most medical doctors prescribe only FDA approved treatments. This alone gives the FDA nearly total control over all treatments. Most people, when the situation arises, go directly to their MD because that is the only way to have the cost of their medical treatment paid by their medical insurance.

The Insurance Companies, the Law, Communication and Freedom of Speech

If any of you visit an average medical doctor expecting a treatment other than drugs and/or surgery, you are living in a fantasy world. Of course there are a few MD's who may prescribe other treatments, but they are hard to find. In my experience and in talking to many others, most medical doctors treat their patients almost exclusively with drugs and surgery. Since most prescription drugs do not TREAT THE CAUSE and therefore DO NOT CURE, there must be a reason why MD's do that. However, the reason why has escaped me for a long time.

At long last, I believe I have finally figured it out; that is the GRASS ROOTS CAUSE of our medical care problem. It has taken many, many years of my own personal experiences, the reading of many books, months of thought and discussions with many others including two medical doctors. I guess I must be a little "slow" in taking so long to figure this out.

When I first began my self treatment for my ALS condition, I really began to learn about the problems with our medical care system. For a long time I wondered about how this could all be happening. Was it a conspiracy? No, I don't think so, but you never know for sure. It could be "conscious parallelism," but then I heard that there was a law that said in effect that only a drug can cure. This seemed to be the perfect explanation. However, I've learned from two medical doctors that is not entirely true because there are no limitations on what a doctor may prescribe. Now it has taken me a long time to figure it out, but I think I have discovered the real answers and there are five:

1. **Drugs and Med School.** Here is where it starts. I believe it all begins in medical school. The medical schools are heavily influenced by Big Pharma. So if all you learn in medical school is about prescription drugs, then how can you do anything else?

2. **Medical Insurance.** There are many different treatments including prescription drugs for many different illnesses. However, only certain treatments are recognized by the medical community AND the medical insurance companies as acceptable treatments. The medical insurance companies will not pay for any other treatments. I don't blame the insurance companies. After all, they should not pay for any treatment that may not work. Most medical doctors know this and in general only recommend those treatments acceptable to the insurance companies.

3. **FDA Approved Treatments.** The FDA approves only those treatments which can be proven to be successful treatments by scientific clinical studies. That generally means only prescription drugs. The drug companies have the money and the people to do this. Although there are many scientific studies of treatments other than prescription drugs, they are rarely submitted to the FDA because they are for natural substances which cannot be patented. For example, you cannot obtain a patent on a vitamin or a mineral. Further, even if you could, no company would ever spend the money for the clinical studies to prove the efficacy of the treatment. There is simply no way to profit.

4. **The Law.** I am dead certain that there must be a law which prevents anyone selling a health product to claim that it can cure. Now don't miss this. Even if they can prove that the product will cure, they dare not make that claim. If they even INSINUATE that their product provides ANY health benefit, the "Medical Mafia" may come after them. This in my opinion is a violation of our Constitutional "Freedom of Speech." Here is a typical disclaimer found on a health care product: "This product has not been evaluated by the Food and Drug Administration. This product is not intended to diagnose,

treat, cure, or prevent disease." Now you and I know that they make that statement to protect themselves. But why in the world would you or I buy the product if it won't treat, cure or help prevent illness? This law must be changed.

This law has far reaching effect on our whole system. This law really prevents anyone selling a health product or providing a health treatment from COMMUNICATING anything positive about the product or treatment unless already approved by the FDA. In other words, if you or I develop a cure for cancer, we are unable to tell anyone about it. Now think about that for a minute. Communication is the whole key to the problem. I believe there are probably hundreds of natural cures that our medical doctors don't know about because communication is restricted by law.

5. **Malpractice Insurance.** Medical doctors are fully aware of the many malpractice claims against medical doctors. For that reason, most doctors prefer to limit their treatments to only those approved by the FDA; that's a fairly safe way to go. Additionally, and after many years of doing this, they become brainwashed to the idea that nothing else will work.

I have rewritten the above many times. It just recently occurred to me that I really don't have to explain why doctors do what they do. I really don't know for sure and all of the above is just my best guess. The one solid fact remains that MOST DOCTORS AVOID ALL NATURAL TREATMENTS IN FAVOR OF PRESCRIPTION DRUGS.

As a result of all this, there is no way to introduce a newly discovered cure other than through the FDA.

Dr. Ignarro was awarded the Nobel Prize in 1998 for his discovery that Nitric Oxide could prevent cardiovascular disease by preventing the buildup of plaque. This treatment involves primarily a diet and the use of a supplement and there is no way you will ever obtain FDA approval for that type of a treatment. So while Dr. Ignarro made a tremendous discovery, it has laid dormant for over ten years. What could have been a great benefit to mankind has been ignored.

Here are two more illustrations of what I mean. It is a well known fact that scurvy is caused by a lack of vitamin C in the diet. It is also well known that adding vitamin C to the diet will CURE scurvy. It is a well known fact that lack of vitamin D (sunshine) is the cause of rickets. It is also well known that taking vitamin D or getting out in the sunshine will cure rickets. These two examples occurred well before the drug companies came into power. If either of these situations would have occurred recently, we would never have a cure for either one. Medical doctors would not have prescribed either vitamin and I'm certain that the drug companies would have developed a drug for their treatment. Do you see now how our medical care system works to PREVENT CURES?

If our medical doctors only prescribe prescription drugs as a treatment for illness, and drugs do not provide a cure, then that means that our medical doctors are unable to provide us with any cures.

Resveratrol is one of the hottest selling supplements on the market today. It will evidently help prevent heart attacks and maybe even cancer. I just read that the drug companies are feverishly working on development of a drug based on Resveratrol and they are spending millions to do it. Now I ask you, how will anyone benefit from this OTHER THAN Big Pharma? Even though it will cost more, our MD's will prescribe it because it will be FDA approved. I think that's a good illustration of how our system works to the advantage of Big Pharma and the disadvantage to the overall health care costs.

All the above is a probable explanation for the fact that we, as a nation, are getting sicker and sicker.

Killing Competition

Here is the first thing you should know about Big Pharma and all competition. IT IS ABSOLUTELY CRITICAL TO BIG PHARMA FOR ALL OF US TO BELIEVE THAT THERE ARE NO CURES AND THAT DRUGS ARE THE ONLY TREATMENT.

This is just one example of what THEY can do. Channel surfing on the TV is one of my pastimes. Two or three years ago, I was surfing and came across an infomercial about coral calcium. Kevin Trudeau was interviewing Dr. Robert Barefoot. I was impressed by their discussion and ordered some coral calcium. They also sent me a pH test kit and one of Barefoot's books "The Calcium Factor: The Scientific Secret of Health and Youth." The company marketing coral calcium enjoyed a great success with their product, BUT WAIT. According to Kevin Trudeau, in his book "Natural Cures 'They' Don't Want You to Know About," the Federal Trade Commission put them out of business overnight. There was no warning and they stormed the main office and confiscated most of their records. According to what I've read, you just don't fight the FTC. They have an over 90% success rate in court. Now this begins to get really interesting. According to Trudeau, they filed their infomercial with the FTC two years prior and with no objections.

It would appear that there could be only two reasons for this action. Either they were saying something wrong like making false claims or the product itself was no good. Neither one seems to be right. If they were making false claims, couldn't the FTC just warn them or tell them to change their infomercial? Apparently this was not done.

It does not appear as though there was any problem with the product, because that same exact product is still on the market as well as many other calcium supplements.

Well then, why do you suppose the FTC did that? Apparently there was no problem with either the infomercial or the product itself. Then what was it? I think it may have been the book they were selling or giving away with every purchase of coral calcium. In the book "The Calcium Factor" by Dr. Barefoot, he provides much information that would make the drug companies very unhappy. Here are two reasons why they would be unhappy:

#1

On the outside cover, Dr. Barefoot states *"Did you know that scientists have found that cancer thrives in an acidic medium, but cannot survive in an alkaline medium?"* If that is true, and I believe it is, that could make all forms of cancer a thing of the past. Wow, imagine that. I have every reason to believe this is true.

#2

Dr. Barefoot in his book tells the story about Dr. Ignas Semmelweis who discovered that washing off the hands would prevent transfer of disease to patients. I told you this story earlier.

You might be thinking that this occurred over a hundred years ago and people have changed. That may be true, but the SYSTEM hasn't. I believe the same thing is going on today, but people don't know that, and that's why I'm writing this book.

*   *   *

Here is another story about the power and influence of the drug companies. On our web site, we provide a Regimen Outline which includes all the treatments, diets, and supplements that I believe are responsible for my being alive today. We don't anymore, but previously we included web sites and phone numbers for some of these supplements. Some of them offered us a commission or a rebate for our referrals. We have always declined to accept any payment. However, we made one exception and that was with Mannatech. When I decided to try their Ambrotose products (a glyconutrient), they offered two prices. There was a lower price for becoming an associate. As an associate, we would receive some small commission for our referrals. However, we lived to regret that.

Apparently the Texas District Attorney filed suit against Mannatech. As a result of the court action, we received a letter from Mannatech telling us that we as an associate must make no claim about health improvement associated with their product. We made many changes on our web site. Then, we received another letter. These letters were rather scary because Mannatech was threatening us with legal action if we did not conform immediately. Again, we made more changes. Finally, after the fourth really demanding letter, we eliminated Mannatech, Ambrotose, glyconutrients and any reference to them from our web site. We also terminated our status as an associate with them.

It became obvious to us that Mannatech was in a state of near panic. I tell you this story for the purpose of letting you know how serious the problem really is. If you want to test this theory all you have to do is this. Develop and market a really good dietary health supplement and become very successful. Then, they will come and put you out of business in a heartbeat. This story has been repeated many, many times in the last few decades.

Here is one more example. The creator of MMS claims to have cured over 75,000 malaria patients in Africa. MMS is used to make chlorine dioxide. It has been declared by one group of scientists as being the most effective killer of pathogens known to man. It is relatively harmless when taken according to instructions. It is so effective IT HAS ALREADY BEEN BANNED IN AUSTRALIA AND CANADA. By the way, it is very inexpensive and could possibly eliminate the need for many antibiotic drugs presently on the market. Big Pharma would not like that.

I just received an e-mail about a major supplier of MMS. The e-mail went on to explain why they were withdrawing MMS from the marketplace effective March 15, 2009. Basically, my interpretation of the e-mail is that they are afraid that some arm of the government such as the FDA may come after them. They are probably right. However, MMS might be the greatest medical discovery since penicillin. The way our system works, our government will simply shut down the sale of a product like this without ever checking it out to see how good or bad it is. If that happened to MMS, it would be a major loss to all of us. I believe chlorine dioxide (made with MMS) can cure a virus including the flu virus. Big Pharma would not be happy about that.

Never underestimate the power of money.

Here is still another story about killing competition. This in my opinion is an indisputable story. A Dr. Robert O. Becker, MD proved that Colloidal Silver can kill many deadly pathogens. It can kill over 650 pathogens. A Dr. Cesar Garcia Ramirez, MD of Mexico is using Colloidal Silver to apparently cure AIDS patients. However, the "powers that be" have for many years now made every effort to restrict the use of Colloidal Silver. They have done this by trying to convince us that Colloidal Silver was INEFFECTIVE. Naturally, they would prefer the use of more expensive and hazardous drugs. According to what I read, the FDA has passed a ruling that prohibits any of us from learning the real truth about Colloidal Silver. Isn't that a good example of a lack of "Freedom of Speech?"

Here is the really funny part. THEY have always told us in the past that Colloidal Silver was not effective. Now they are telling us that Colloidal Silver is so effective that they don't want it to get in our water supplies and kill all bacteria. Isn't that a strange turn around? That is exactly the opposite of what they were saying before. Doesn't that tell us that they are trying to hide the real truth?

There is a new drug on the market that the drug companies are trying desperately to convince us is a life saver. They claim that it may prevent cervical cancer. Now let's stop right there. Did you say that some drug could PREVENT an illness? Well, take notice that they say "it may" prevent cancer of a certain type. This is only my opinion, but I believe it is TOTALLY INSANE to take a TOXIC drug or anything toxic to PREVENT an illness. Toxin means poison. Every toxic drug has horrible possible side effects. Side effects can include death as we have already discussed. It seems to me that you simply trade one POSSIBLE illness for another possible illness. Does that really make sense?

This is what they said in an article in the "The Desert Sun" on 9-14-08. The clinical study involved 15,000 women for two years. Of the group not receiving the vaccination, nineteen women developed PRECANCEROUS lesions because of HPV infection. NONE of the vaccination group developed precancerous lesions. Apparently NONE OF THE WOMEN in either group developed cancer. Now, do you understand what they first said? They said not one person developed cancer. From all that I've read, there is no evidence that the HPV virus causes cancer. They only suspect that it does. Well, in my book, suspect is not enough. From the information I have gathered, there are over 100 types of cancer. This vaccine may only help in two types of cancer. What about the other more than 98? Does that mean we need another 50 or more vaccines? I don't think vaccinations are the answer to our cancer problem.

While we're talking about vaccinations, let's get down to the nitty-gritty. The question is: Do we really need vaccinations? I'm not sure, maybe yes or maybe no. But, we may be going down the wrong path and let me tell you why I say that.

They say that the 1918 flu pandemic killed an estimated 50 million people worldwide. Wow, that's a lot of people. BUT, what's really interesting is the fact that LESS THAN 5% of the deaths occurred within three days. That would indicate that those few deaths were the only ones DIRECTLY caused by the flu virus. Medical scientists believe that most of the deaths were due to pneumonia caused by secondary bacterial infections. Many of these deaths occurred seven to ten days from onset and many died after two weeks.

Another interesting fact is that in some households the entire family died, while in other homes only one or two died. The obvious conclusion is that those survivors must have had better immune systems. No doubt there were many more people who survived the flu pandemic than those who died.

According to a recent newspaper article, many people are refusing vaccinations for their children and hundreds of thousands will be going to school this year without them. Many parents are apparently learning that the vaccinations may not be worth the risk.

My conclusion is that we should be helping people boost their immune systems rather than using vaccinations. There's more information in later chapters about the immune system.

I have never had a flu vaccination other than perhaps when I was in the Army. I've only had the flu once or twice. The last time was over 30 years ago. I've heard many people say they came down with the flu right after they had a flu shot. Here is the problem the way I see it. Every year the flu epidemic kills many people, but every year the flu is caused by a different virus. Usually the flu shot they give you this year would be formulated to treat last year's virus. Obviously, that doesn't always work. I personally think this is another fraud.

The way I see it, getting a flu shot and expecting to avoid the flu is just like jumping off your garage roof holding an umbrella.

Swine Influenza

Here we are on May 1, 2009, and I still haven't finished writing this book. Now along comes the *'pig flu.'* I simply must give you my thoughts about this so-called flu epidemic. I'm predicting right now that this will not become an epidemic, and it's a long way from becoming a pandemic. OK, I was wrong. It has developed into a pandemic. But, that's only a technicality because the common cold is also a pandemic and it does not kill very many people. The swine flu has not yet killed even 1% of the number of people who die every year from the regular flu.

Here's what we know about the flu. Every year about 36,000 people DIE from the flu in the U.S.A. Millions more get the flu and do not die. In 1918, they had a flu pandemic that killed about 50 million people worldwide. As of today, no U.S. resident has died from the swine flu. Incidentally, 90% of those who died in 1918 DID NOT die DIRECTLY from the flu. Over 90% of them died from secondary infections of bacteria. If that happened today, we have antibiotics to prevent that from reoccurring.

Now here is the big question: WHAT IN THE HELL IS ALL THE BIG FUSS ABOUT? The news media is all over this like white on rice and causing a near panic throughout the country, and yet this flu is milder than the normal flu. The only thing different about the swine flu is that it is a new strain, but so what? They don't have a real cure for any flu.

In 1976, we had a similar flu outbreak. President Gerald Ford wanted to give everyone in the whole country flu shots. Well, guess what happened? They did not do that, and very few people died from that flu. Interestingly more people died from the FLU SHOTS than those who died from the flu.

The above is what I believe are the facts, but now I want to move into the world of FICTION. This is all my imagination.

What if this was all deliberate? You might think my imagination has gone wild, but you should see some logic in my story. Here is what could have happened. Two top executives of a Big Pharma company are discussing the current economy and their reduced sales. They also recognize that many people are avoiding their annual flu shots and avoiding vaccinations for their children. The two executives are concerned about what to do. One suggests "Maybe we should create a flu epidemic just to teach the public a lesson and do it with a flu virus that has never been seen before." The other exec says "Yes but we don't want to kill a lot of people doing it."

If I was totally unscrupulous and the head of a large drug company, I would do it in a heartbeat. I believe it would also be a great idea to begin the flu in a foreign country where it could spread rapidly to the U.S.A. Mexico would be perfect. I would even consider introducing a less minor flu in the U.S. In any event, one or both flu viruses would be mild and less contagious.

I am not suggesting for a minute that Big Pharma is responsible for this. However, you must know that they are fully capable of doing something like this. My point is that you should know that and you should be very suspicious. You can never trust anyone too much.

Now folks, here is the latest I have read about the source of the swine flu. A man who has studied germ evolution for 40 years has published a paper on his theory about the source of the swine flu. He said that the H1N1 virus was probably man-made and caused by human error. If you match that to my above theory, you may draw a very interesting conclusion.

This story does not prove anything, but you might find it interesting. When I was a kid back in the 1930's and 1940's, I never had the flu and I never knew of anyone who had the flu. It may have been around, but I simply did not know about it. Nowadays, they have a flu epidemic every year that kills thousands of people. I cannot help but wonder what has changed and who may have caused the change.

There was one drug in 2004 that studies showed that it doubled your risk of a heart attack. According to what I read, the company knew all about this before it was approved and covered it up. While it was on the market, it is estimated that it killed (murdered) 139,000 people. How can they sleep at night?

Now here's one about another drug. You may not believe this one, so I will quote from the article of 2-23-08 in the "Los Angeles Times." The sub-headline read and I quote:

"The FDA approves the drug's use despite a lack of evidence that it extends patients' lives."

Now get this, we are talking about the use of a $100,000 a year drug for breast cancer. Another quote from the articles says *"Research shows the drug slows the progress of breast cancer tumors by more than five months but does not extend patients' lives."* Remember, all you gals reading this, this drug also has significant side effects including some deaths. Also, the FDA advisory panel voted against approval, but the FDA approved it anyway. Wow!

Never underestimate the power of money. The drug companies have a lot of money.

This was the headline for an article in the "Los Angeles Times" 11-10-07: *"Merck's Vioxx tactic pays off."* The subheading said *"After initially fighting all claims, it works out a $4.85 billion deal that could limit its liability."* Apparently this all came about from a study that showed the drug doubled the risk of heart attacks and strokes.

Most of us have a great fear of cancer. The drug companies know they can sell us almost anything because of that fear. One of the major problems with our medical care system today is that the MD's believe almost anything the drug companies tell them AND the patients believe anything the doctor says. In fact, one state governor wanted to pass a law requiring all women of a certain age to take a new cancer prevention drug.

Now that in itself is another totally insane idea. We should not pass laws forcing people to do anything about their own personal health that they might not want to do. To begin with, they offer no solid evidence of what the drug may do. According to what I've read, OVER 100 WOMEN HAVE ALREADY DIED from this new drug which was introduced only about two years ago. How would you feel if your wife or daughter dropped dead from taking this drug and you later found out that this drug was unnecessary? In my opinion, it is unnecessary because there are other precautions which may be taken that are a more effective way of prevention. This makes me really wonder about how little they care about human life.

I have saved the best two stories for the last of this chapter. You will really love both of them: The Cholesterol Story and The Chelation Story:

The Cholesterol Story

About 40 years ago in the 1960's, "Time/Life" published a magazine all about heart attacks (remember, I'm older than dirt). This special publication discussed four major causes. One - smoking. Two - sedentary lifestyle. Three - diet. Now remember I'm an old guy and doing this all from memory. I simply cannot recall the fourth item. However, in the diet section they discussed cholesterol. At that time we were just beginning to suspect that high cholesterol might be a problem. HOWEVER, it was a consensus among the medical doctors at that time that Triglycerides were of far more significance than cholesterol. Now, for the rest of the story:

THERE IS NO SIGNIFICANT EVIDENCE THAT HIGH CHOLESTEROL HAS ANYTHING TO DO WITH THE CAUSE OF HEART ATTACKS AND STROKES.

Actually here's what happened. There was a major study called the "Framingham Study" that initially indicated that cholesterol was the problem. Thus the cholesterol story began. HOWEVER, a short time later they apologized for their mistake and stated clearly that they were wrong about cholesterol. The apology or correction came too late and was almost totally ignored.

For years now, medical doctors have relied on high blood pressure to be an indication of a circulatory problem. Based on what I've read and my own opinion, I think that is still true. However, many doctors are prescribing drugs to lower your cholesterol even if you do not have high blood pressure. Does that make sense to you? I don't think so.

Let me try to prove my point beyond any reasonable doubt with the following facts:

Fact One. There is a TV commercial that I've seen a number of times by one of the drug companies advertising their statin drug. In very small print and for only a few seconds, they say that their drug *"HAS NOT BEEN SHOWN TO PREVENT HEART ATTACKS AND STROKES."*

Can you believe that? They are admitting that their drug will not do for you what you believe it will do.

Now I ask you, why in the world would anyone in their right mind take the drug? Why in their right mind would any MD prescribe the drug?

Fact Two. It is estimated that about 40 million people in the U.S. are taking a statin drug to lower their cholesterol and believing they are preventing a heart attack or stoke. The total sales of all statin drugs taken to lower cholesterol is estimated at approximately $50 billion a year.

Fact Three. More than half of the heart attack victims have normal or low cholesterol.

Fact Four. The company who makes another of the statin drugs makes the following statement in their advertising: *"(Their drug) is FDA-approved to reduce the risk of heart attack and stroke in patients, etc."* Now, if I read that correctly, they do not say that their drug actually reduces heart attacks and strokes. They say that their drug was "APPROVED" to do that, but it does not say that it actually does that. I think that's very clever. Kudos to their advertising department.

Fact Five. It is probably common knowledge that plaque in your arteries is the real culprit causing heart attacks. An article in the "Los Angeles Times" on 1-15-08 said in a subtitle *"A study funded by the firms that make the cholesterol blocker says it doesn't help fight arterial plaque."*

If lowering cholesterol by taking the statin drugs really prevented heart attacks, then there should have been a massive decline in the number of heart attacks. THAT JUST HAS NOT HAPPENED and they have been selling these drugs for about TWENTY FIVE YEARS. This is probably the biggest single drug success story of all time. It may also be the biggest fraud of all time.

Sometimes statistical evidence is not as meaningful as one human experience. Here is a letter published in the "Los Angeles Times" 6-22-09 and I find it very interesting and thought provoking: *"In less than two years on Lipitor, I went from being able to climb the ancient temples at Angkor Wat, Cambodia, to being almost unable to walk to my mailbox. I felt like I had the flu all the time. I had pains in my fingers, arms, shoulders, hips, legs and feet. My doctor took me off Lipitor. Four days later, I could move my fingers again."*

There was an article in the "Los Angeles Times" 4-7-08. Here is the sub-headline: *"Some doctors stand by Vytorin after a surprising study; others question if cholesterol matters at all."* The following quote is the first paragraph of the article: *"The cholesterol drug did absolutely everything it was supposed to do—except for demonstrably improving the health of the people who took it."* Now, folks, that's really some conclusion. In my words, the drug is totally useless and of course dangerous.

Lowering total cholesterol may not be the answer. IF lowering total cholesterol had any appreciable effect on lowering heart attacks, it is offset by increased risk of cancer according to a clinical study several years ago. The body produces 80% of our cholesterol. Cholesterol is necessary for good health. However, you have HDL cholesterol (good) and LDL cholesterol (bad). You do not want to lower good cholesterol. You may want to reduce bad cholesterol, but this is probably BEST DONE BY DIET. Triglycerides may be far more significant than cholesterol. High Triglycerides is a true health concern and may be far more serious than high cholesterol. This too may best be treated by diet.

The above "Cholesterol Story" was written about ten days ago and now (11-10-08), the "Los Angeles Times" had an article on EXPANDING the use of statin drugs. Can you believe that?

Here is the sub-headline: *"Statin drugs can cut cardiac and stroke risks in people with normal cholesterol levels, researchers say."* However, the rest of the article does not prove that to me; and guess who paid for and conducted the study? None other than the drug company who sells one of the most expensive statin drugs. Their drug sells for $3.45 a day, but generic statin drugs sell for less than $1.00.

The study involved people with NORMAL cholesterol and the article claimed that the drug lowered the risk of death from heart disease by 20%. Now, I find that hard to believe, because there's no evidence in the real world that statin drugs do that for people with high cholesterol. How in the world will the same drug lower the death rate in people with normal cholesterol? That's not logical. They also claim that their new drug could prevent 50,000 heart attacks, strokes and deaths each year. Then they go on to say that 120 people would have to take the new drug for two years to prevent one heart attack, stroke or death. Wow, imagine that? Over 100 people have to suffer the horrible side effects in order to prevent one heart attack or stroke or death. Again, that does not add up to me. Maybe I'm pessimistic about drugs, but remember who paid for the study. I just don't buy it.

I have a report written by a doctor about one company's statin drug study. The report states that their drug did reduce the number of heart attacks of those taking the drug vs. the placebo. HOWEVER, the actual number of FATAL heart attacks was higher by 50% for those taking the drug vs. those taking the placebo. Now, that should just rattle your cage like a 9.0 earthquake. It sure does mine.

The Nitric Oxide (NO) and Dr. Ignarro Story

Here is one more smashing story about cardiovascular health that relates to the above Cholesterol Story and one more reason why we DO NOT need all those drugs to lower cholesterol.

Dr. Louis Ignarro was awarded the Nobel Prize in Medicine in 1998 for his discovery that fish, fruits and vegetables could prevent and/or cure heart problems. Now before you think that's nutty, let me tell you the FULL story. What I said is true, but there's more to it than that. Dr. Ignarro was really awarded the Nobel Prize for discovering that Nitric Oxide (NO) is a molecule that may prevent and cure many diseases including heart disease. But, the best way to increase your body's NO is by eating more fruits, vegetables and fish. Additionally, he recommends taking an NO supplement, 30 minutes of exercise daily, and drink plenty of pure water.

That was over ten years ago and to the best of my knowledge medical doctors have not stopped prescribing drugs. Now I have a really serious question for you: Why are doctors not using this information on NO? It seems to me to be simply logical that we should take advantage of this valuable information about treating all illness and especially heart disease. If someone is awarded a Nobel Prize for something, you would think that the "something" must have tremendous value. How can we then ignore it? It's not logical.

Here is how I think it should work using the above as an example. Prescription drugs should not be used exclusively. Drugs and natural therapies should be used in combination. Let's say you have a heart attack and you are rushed to the E.R. The doctors should logically use drugs to save your life because they work faster. But then, I think it would be logical to begin as soon as practical a natural treatment such as Dr. Ignarro recommends. This is only logical because the heart drugs probably will never cure the problem.

Here is another question for you. How does a treatment such as this one of Dr. Ignarro ever become a mainstream treatment by most doctors?

If you want more information, visit the web site:

www.drignarro.com

Never underestimate the power of money.

Well, that's the end of my Cholesterol Story for now.

The Chelation Story

The beginning of the Chelation story goes all the way back to World War II; that's right, Chelation treatment has been around for well over 50 years. It all started during World War II when we were building hundreds, maybe thousands, of ocean going vessels or ships. We won the war partially because we simply out produced the enemy. There were thousands of workers employed in the ship building yards. A lot of Lead is used in the construction of ships. As a result, many workers developed Lead poisoning. The government asked the drug companies to develop a treatment.

They learned that German doctors had already developed EDTA for the treatment of Lead poisoning. So, the FDA approved EDTA. EDTA by IV must be done by a doctor. EDTA is now available in other forms including suppositories and liquid. The EDTA enters your bloodstream and while traveling through your body it chelates (binds) with Lead and carries it out of the body through the normal elimination process. A funny thing happened. Not really funny, but strange. It was observed that all the workers being treated with EDTA Chelation had a lower heart attack rate than normal. How about that sports fans? This information has been ignored and suppressed for all these years.

I read somewhere that in Australia a patient is required to have Chelation treatment before any heart surgery. I also read that in Sweden they had a group of people waiting for heart surgery and while they waited they were given Chelation treatments. By the time their surgery date came up, they did not need it.

Most doctors do not offer Chelation by IV and I'm not really sure why. Apparently the medical establishment does not approve of it.

However, there is a non-profit organization called American College of Advancement in Medicine (ACAM). One of their founding doctors said; *"Our group has verifiable medical data on more than 500,000 patients who have received EDTA Chelation therapy since the early fifties. Over 85% of those treated received at least some benefit; more than 20% who had been given up for dead by orthodox physicians, are still around and enjoying life. Adverse reactions are practically nonexistent. There have been fewer than 30 EDTA-related deaths in comparison with the more than 18,000 deaths as a direct consequence of bypass surgery in the same period."*

My personal medical doctor provides Chelation treatments for patients. He has one large room with about ten large comfortable reclining chairs for patients undergoing the two to three hour IV drip. I have been in that room once or twice a week for many weeks during the last five or six years. All in all, I've probably spent one or two hundred hours in there. Often during the Chelation treatments patients share their experiences in a group discussion. I have only heard praise about the Chelation treatment. Many people have said that Chelation was the smartest thing they've ever done for their health. Everyone seems to have lower blood pressure as a result of the treatments.

There is not the slightest doubt in my mind about whether or not this is an effective treatment. It may be the single best treatment for your heart and circulatory system that exists today. If more people knew about this, and if more doctors would use it, we could probably reduce the number of deaths from heart attacks significantly. Why don't we do it?

Those last three stories are verifiable and should prove beyond any doubt that our medical system is not only UNREASONABLY EXPENSIVE and INEFFICIENT, but also CORRUPT BEYOND BELIEF.

American history tells us to remember three events:

1. Remember the Maine.
2. Remember the Alamo.
3. Remember Pearl Harbor.

Someday we will look back and remember two more:

4. Remember Big Tobacco.
5. Remember Big Pharma. The big daddy of them all.

WHO KNOWS WHAT EVIL LURKS IN THE HEARTS OF MEN? That statement pretty well sums up this chapter. That is from an old radio show in the 1930's and '40's called "The Shadow." The above statement was followed with *"THE SHADOW KNOWS."*

Where is "The Shadow" when we really need him?

Natural Antibiotics

There are several NATURAL antibiotics, but two of them are outstanding. I say that because they are not true antibiotics. The word "biotic" comes from a word that means "life." So, antibiotic means anti-life. All antibiotic drugs that I know about are truly anti-life. BUT, Colloidal Silver and chlorine dioxide are SELECTIVE. That is, they are like the Lone Ranger, and they only kill the bad guys and do no harm to all the cells in your body who wear white hats.

The doctors have been using far too many antibiotics for many years now and the result is the bad bugs have mutated and become resistant to them. Not even penicillin works on them now.

Here is just one example: MRSA, or methicillin-resistant staphylococcus aureus, is a deadly flesh-eating drug-resistant "super pathogen." This bug or pathogen is now responsible for an estimated 94,000 life-threatening infections and 18,650 deaths annually. Incidentally, that's more than the number of deaths caused by AIDS. So, evidently our drug antibiotics are not working. My ex-wife died from this after a lengthy illness including more than 20 separate surgeries over a three-year period.

In the 1970's, a Dr. Robert O. Becker, MD, discovered a cure for MRSA. Not only that, his cure healed every "incurable" infection that they brought to him. Since then, this information has been SUPPRESSED. However, several recent studies have re-established the fact that Colloidal Silver can cure infectious disease, probably better than any drug antibiotic. That's why it's been suppressed.

Chlorine dioxide may do the same thing as Colloidal Silver, and based on my personal experience with both, chlorine dioxide acts faster. There's more info on both of these amazing elements in later chapters.

OK, now we are at the end of this chapter and you might wonder if I'm mad at Big Pharma? Well, the answer is *"Hell yes."* Remember, it was a prescription drug that almost killed me and then the doctors told me I was on my own. Wouldn't you be mad when you woke up paralyzed?

You should never complain about something, unless you have a suggestion for a better way. My conclusion about Big Pharma is that they use their billions of dollars to influence. Recently the Chinese EXECUTED the head of their FDA for bribery. Clever those Chinese. Do you think that would be appropriate here?

I hope you don't mind, but I must remind you once again. This was all predicted by Dr. Benjamin Rush, the only medical doctor to sign the U.S. Constitution.

There is an old axiom that goes something like this *"Fool me once shame on you, fool me twice shame on me."* Most of us continue to visit our medical doctors even though they do not offer a cure for most of our illnesses. Should that be a *"Shame on us?"*

Here is one more thought for the end of this chapter and don't miss this. This is one you really should contemplate. Imagine for a moment that someone other than a medical doctor is describing to you the benefits and the possible side effects of a pill. The person is telling you that the pill WILL NOT cure you and then the person tells you of all the horrible side effects such as going blind, losing your hearing, and on and on, and that includes possibly being fatal. Now ask yourself; do the benefits REALLY outweigh the risk and would you REALLY buy this product and use it? My thought is that you would not. I think we put way too much trust in the doctor and completely overlook the possible side effects.

Is anyone really listening to the warnings about major side effects of prescription drugs in their TV commercials?

One of the statements I hear often in the drug commercials is something like this: *"This drug may not be suitable for everyone."* Can you imagine that?

"Not suitable." Actually, I think that is a CLASSIC statement. Maybe better yet, that is a COLLOSSAL UNDERSTATEMENT. Since thousands of people die every year from prescription drugs, I don't think their drugs are "suitable" for anyone, but that's only my opinion. Do medical doctors really question their patient's "suitability" when they prescribe a drug? I don't think so.

It appears to me that Big Pharma is ONLY interested in more and more profits and they don't give a damn about the effect of their products on our lives. Remember, I've been in a wheelchair for well over ten years AS A RESULT OF A SINGLE PRESCRIPTION DRUG.

Again, all this was predicted by Dr. Benjamin Rush.

I BELIEVE THERE ARE NO INCURABLE ILLNESSES.

CHAPTER 9

OUR BELIEF SYSTEMS

I know that OUR BELIEF SYSTEMS represent one of our BIGGEST PROBLEMS WITH HEALTH CARE. Real cures are forced into hiding by all the false information, and our belief system does the rest.

Here is just one simple example of what I mean. If your medical doctor tells you to go home and die because there's nothing he can do, most people BELIEVE that and follow his directions. However, a drowning man will fight vigorously to maintain life, even grasping for straws. What is the difference in these two situations? The difference is our belief system. Now, the drowning man was not told by the doctor that there was no hope. For that reason, I would like to spend a little of your time analyzing our belief systems.

In trying to understand more about our belief systems, I conducted a little experiment recently. I asked two of my friends, separately of course, about Big Foot. I told them I thought Big Foot could be real. Each of them answered in their own way, but their basic reactions were the same. They were appalled that I would BELIEVE such a thing and each of them proceeded to tell me that Big Foot cannot be. I never got one word in edgewise. When they finished telling my why that could not be, our discussion ended.

Now I don't know whether or not Big Foot exists. But, I am open to that possibility because I watched a one-hour TV documentary which included a great deal of EVIDENCE that Big Foot may exist. For the sake of this discussion, it does not matter whether Big Foot exists or not. The point is my two friends were not open-minded to any possibility that Big Foot exists. Their attitudes were like "Don't confuse me with the facts, my mind is already made up." I am not being critical of them because we are all the same way to one degree or another, and that includes me. The point is we should not be so convinced about something we only BELIEVE in and don't really KNOW. That kind of thinking can hurt us, especially when it comes to health care. We should be open-minded to THOUGHTS and/or EVIDENCE.

Before we go any further, we should define the three words—THINK—BELIEVE—KNOW. Many of us use these words interchangeably, but each has a very different meaning. Which one of these three words you select usually depends on the amount of evidence of the real truth.

Think

This word is used when we have limited information, and we are really not certain.

Believe

When we use this word, it usually means we have a little more evidence on the subject, and we are a little more certain about the truth. However, we are still not SURE. That's what this chapter is all about. To believe or not to believe; that is the question.

Know

When we use the word know, that should mean that we are totally convinced, beyond any reasonable doubt.

Here is an example of what I mean. When we say we BELIEVE in God, that is saying a lot more than just that we THINK there is a God. However, we don't use the word KNOW, because there is limited evidence of God. Believing is the correct word.

So, Eric, *"Why all this grammar lesson?"* My answer is that I will be using these words very carefully in this book and I want you to know that. Remember, this chapter is all about BELIEVING.

Brainwashing

Another word that we must define is "brainwashing." Brainwashing is a method of altering someone's belief system by repeat, repeat, and more repeat. If we hear something often enough, we will tend to believe it even without facts or evidence.

We should learn to question our own beliefs by asking ourselves what do we really know about the facts or have we been brainwashed on the subject? Probably the best example is "cholesterol." We have literally been brainwashed about cholesterol for several decades now and without any evidence or facts. I've already told you all the facts about cholesterol and I hope you are now convinced that you are a victim of brainwashing. SO, you must remember what I first told you in the very beginning of this book. You should not automatically believe EVERYTHING your doctor tells you. You should learn to look for the facts and/or evidence.

When we are first born, we come into this world with a clean slate; that is we KNOW nothing. During the first 10 years or so, we accept and believe all that we are told without question. These BELIEFS become fairly rigid. People do not like to change their beliefs about anything that they have already learned, whether it be right or wrong. This also happens all through our lives. Anything we have learned a long time ago becomes almost a permanent fixture. It is very difficult to change someone's mind even with a lot of evidence. I remember when I was very young, I thought teachers, policemen, and ministers were all perfect people. Then later, it was difficult for me to accept the fact that they are not all perfect.

It is important for you and I to understand our belief systems as they effect us as PATIENTS and also effect our understanding of our MEDICAL DOCTORS.

History has shown that our beliefs on a given subject can be wrong. Just because the mainstream thinkers say that it is so, that doesn't make it correct. It was only about 500 years ago that everyone in the world BELIEVED that the world was flat. That's one example of where the mainstream thinkers were wrong.

Here are a few more examples of what I mean:

Movies

Prior to 1930, we had only silent movies. There was no talking or any other sound. Someone, I'm not sure who, invented sound motion pictures or "talkies" as they were called then. The company with this new idea tried to sell it to every major studio in Hollywood and there were no buyers. Can you believe that? These people were so set on their pre-established ideas, that they could not conceive the value of this new idea. They finally sold the idea to a new up-coming film studio and you know the rest of the story.

Clocks and Watches

For years, the watch manufacturers in Switzerland had a corner on the market for quality watches and clocks. If it had a "Swiss Movement," it was quality stuff. One of the Swiss watch companies developed the digital clock and digital watch. They could not see the value of the digital clock/watch and felt that it would never amount to anything. Boy, were they wrong or what? Obviously, the digital clock/watch did not fit in with their pre-established beliefs, so they sold the idea to a Japanese company. You know the rest of the story. Do you know what the total sales of all digital clocks and watches have been since then? Well, I'm not going to tell you because I don't know either. You can rest assured that it is in the billions of dollars. This is just another example of our human frailty regarding the acceptance or denial of new ideas. Don't fall into that trap.

Brain Cells

Here is a more recent example. Prior to the mid 1980's, the medical community was convinced that human brain cells were not reproduced. I guess that meant that when they all died, you did too. Now we know that's wrong. As brain cells wear out, they are constantly being reproduced at the rate of about 10,000 daily.

U.S. Patent Office

At one time about a hundred years ago, Congress wanted to close the U.S. Patent Office. Why on earth would they want to do that? Well, believe it or not, they thought all the possible new ideas or inventions had already been invented. *"Eric, are you kidding?"* No I'm not; that's the truth. That's about the epitome of denying or non-acceptance of new ideas.

Politics and Religion

There's an old axiom that says *"Never involve yourself in a discussion of politics or religion."* There's a good reason for that. You should probably avoid discussing any topic which you are not willing to entertain the other person's point of view. Each of us has our own belief system and for most of us our beliefs are set in concrete. To violate this rule, you risk losing a friend.

Here is an example of how firm our beliefs can be and how they may be carried too far. Charlie was a retired marine helicopter pilot. He was offered the opportunity to fly the Presidential helicopter. In other words, the President of the U.S.A. selected Charlie to be his pilot. Charlie refused. You want to know why? The President was a Republican and Charlie was a Democrat. I may have that reversed, but that's not the point. Charlie said he would never be a pilot for a man representing the "other" party. Well, I think that's really stupid. We are all Americans first.

Believing the Medical Doctor

One of our pre-established BELIEFS is that the medical doctor is the last word. Let me point out that most medical doctors believe that too. We are literally brainwashed right from the beginning about THE DOCTOR. When we are children and we get sick, mother takes us to the MD. Most mothers never would dream of doing anything else. Consequently, we continue doing that without question. However, as difficult as it may be, we should begin to question that.

Here's the point of all this. If your doctor tells you that you have some incurable disease, then you need to be open-minded to alternative treatments and alternative health practitioners. THERE ARE NO INCURABLE DISEASES. Did you know that 60% of all cancer patients seek alternative treatments? Obviously, they are less than impressed with the medical doctors' treatments. If you think that only medical doctors can help you, then you have a problem with your belief system.

Abe Lincoln is credited with the following statement:

"You can fool all of the people some of the time, some of the people all of the time, but you cannot fool all of the people all of the time."

Well, I know he was so right, because that is what's going on now. Most all of us are being fooled now and have been fooled for a long time. We've been fooled because they don't tell us that drugs don't cure. They don't tell us or advertise the fact that there are over 80 diseases for which they have no cure. Do you really think that is logical in this the 21st century? Through DNA analysis we can prove who your father is and who your mother is, but we can't cure most of our illnesses. Let me tell you how dumb that is.

There are only a few general CAUSES of illness.

You can die from no food, no water, or no air. If that happens, you don't need a doctor to tell you why. You can also get sick and die from food lacking in NUTRITIONAL VALUE.

You can get sick and die from POLLUTED air, water and/or food.

You can also get sick and/or die from infectious diseases caused by pathogens.

Now again, in general, those are the only causes of illness that I know of other than physical injury. I mean what else is there?

If you develop some illness from a large dose of something toxic, your doctor will be able to figure it out. Probably you will already know too. However, if you develop an illness such as cancer or Alzheimer's, you may not know the cause. There should be no mystery. Cancer and Alzheimer's are both illnesses that primarily occur in older people. This means that the cause is probably a lack of proper nutrition and/or exposure to a toxin or toxins over a long period of time. The length of time is the obvious clue.

This is an over simplification, but we do know the cause of every illness and the cause is NOT a lack of prescription drugs in our system. Well anyway, that's the process I went through to figure out the cause of my ALS condition. Then I figured out how to treat the cause, and that's why I'm alive today.

We live in a mobile home park for people age 55 and over. We knew when we moved in here that we would soon see many of them pass away; that was expected. What was not expected was that I would know how their lives may have been extended. I have seen so many people die in the last few years of totally preventable illnesses. This is sad and very frustrating. What is truly interesting is that I am unable to help them. Although I am a walking miracle having survived a terminal illness, that does not convince my neighbors and personal friends of anything.

We have published a book about my experience and protocol. It has sold over 12,000 copies as of August 2008. There are only 5,000 or 6,000 new ALS patients each year in the U.S.A. Many people have written to me to let me know they have followed my protocol and they are improving. Yet, again, my friends and relatives and neighbors ignore anything I offer. This is very frustrating to watch people die, know what could save them, and yet be unable to help. The good side of this is that I'm writing this book to help people. It finally dawned on me that the major hurdle to helping others is that they must realize that we have a problem with our medical care system; and that, my friends, takes more than a few words from me or anyone else. That's what made me realize that I must write a book because it would take a MASSIVE amount of information to change their belief.

This is a story about 80 year old Dorothy who is an intelligent woman and a retired RN. Dorothy is also very healthy and active in sports. She developed cancer in one lung and the doctor recommended surgery. Following a successful surgery, they suggested chemotherapy to prevent any reoccurrence. A health-nut friend named Eric again warned her about the dangers of chemotherapy. She did it anyway. A few doses of the chemo almost killed her. It put her in the hospital and they removed her appendix.

A year or so later, she developed a small cancer in her other lung. Again the friend warned about drug treatments and provided her with ample information about alternative treatments. Again she went with the doctor's recommendation. The doctor recommended a new drug that would not cure the cancer but it MIGHT add a year or so to her life. Same thing happened. These are her exact words: "*The drug he suggested for "prolonging" my life damn near killed me—I spent two days in the hospital trying to get my electrolytes back to normal. Liquid diarrhea for ten days is not good.*"

It was about 5:00 A.M. the other morning when I woke up and began thinking about Dorothy and her cancer. It is so hard for me to understand why people sometimes just give up and won't try even the simplest thing. I asked Dorothy the other day if she had given up. She answered no. However, to the best of my knowledge, she is doing nothing about her cancer. I think what's happened is that a person gets so discouraged following the doctors treatments that they just do not want to try anymore.

Dorothy is showing interest in alternative treatments and has read two books about treating cancer with better food. When I asked her about following some form of a diet, she said in effect it was too much trouble. I would bet you though that if the doctor called her and said he had another treatment for her, she would do it in a minute. My conclusion is, that by the time we are adults, we have been fooled many times and we just do not want to be fooled again. Therefore, we are reluctant to really try anything that we are not absolutely certain of. After all, we do not want to appear foolish. *"Eric, do you mean that people would rather die than try?"* I guess so; what other answer is there?

Now folks, take note that the average cost for all cancer treatment by doctors, drugs and hospitals is about $330,000 per cancer patient. Incidentally, there are no refunds if the treatment does not work.

In the above story, there were three events: lung surgery, chemo and a life extending drug. Now, let's divide the average cost of cancer treatment by three. This will not be accurate, but it will suffice for the purpose of this discussion. OK? If so, let's say that each of the three events costs $110,000. In the first event, the RN did benefit so the cost is appropriate and it was well earned by the doctor. In other words, she got what she paid for.

In the second and third events, she received no benefits at all. In fact, she lost. Now, here's my main point. NO REFUND. If you hired a contractor to remodel your house, and he did not do what you hoped for, you would not pay the bill. RIGHT? But in the case of medical care, the medical doctors, hospitals and the drug companies keep their money anyway. Now you 'gotta' think about that for a minute. Does that seem right? I don't think so. Our system gives them the right to charge whatever they want, whether or not the patient benefits. That just does not sit right with me.

Make note of the fact that the AMA functions much like a union for all medical doctors. Also note that there are no refunds when the doctor fails miserably.

Now back to our belief system.

We are so brainwashed about the medical doctor being the only game in town that we fail to even consider alternatives. Dorothy, from the above story, and I have had many discussions about alternative treatments. I've also provided her with "mucho" information about alternative cancer treatments. She generally agrees with me, but when the chips are down, she will not try any treatment other than what THE DOCTOR RECOMMENDS. I think I know why.

People who have worked in the medical care system a long time are so brainwashed they simply believe that all else just does not work and they just will not even try it. I think there's another element too. Dorothy is an older woman, and has already survived longer than she expected to. She simply may not want to put forth the effort to live any longer. Perhaps there's even a third element. Most people who believe in God, also believe that God is directing or in control of their lives. So, at the first sign of adversity in their health, many people think that God is telling them that it's time to give up and die. I don't believe that. I do not believe that God MICRO-MANAGES our lives.

Here is one more possible explanation. Dorothy has been through three bouts with cancer treatment; the surgery, the chemo, and the life-extending drug. Those three experiences have no doubt seriously damaged her faith. That's gotta be a tough row to hoe. Remember, my doctors told me to go home and die well over a decade ago. If I would have given up then, I would not be helping people like I am today and I would not be writing this book. I believe there is a time to give up, but don't give up too soon.

Conclusion about Beliefs

One of the main reasons we have this medical care problem in our country is because too many of us believe our medical doctors are like God and we believe EVERYTHING they tell us. BUT, your doctor has no cures other than surgery. Medical doctors use only drugs and most drugs do not cure. Therefore, if you get really sick, and you are looking for a CURE, you must be OPEN MINDED to alternatives other than your MD.

Never be a "know-it-all."

"It's what you learn after your think you 'know it all' that really counts."

I really feel sorry for the person we call a "know-it-all," because they will probably never learn anything new. They simply do not have an open mind. I believe we should never be so closed minded that we refuse to CONSIDER other information. Here is a story that illustrates what you can learn even if you think you may know it all.

Glenna and I love trout fishing, especially in the High Sierras in Middle Eastern California. About seven years ago, we were fishing on the shore of Rock Creek Lake. As we approached the shoreline of our favorite spot, we realized that all the good spots were occupied. We like this lake because it is the only place I can drive my three-wheel electric scooter right up to the water's edge and enjoy fishing. After a while, two men told us they were leaving their spot and that we could have it. One of the men took a real interest in us and helped Glenna. He proceeded to tell her all about how to fish and even helped her rig up her line. He very carefully explained how he did the rigging with a bubble. All the time he's talking, I'm thinking of what I might say to him. Something like this, *"Hey, pal, I don't need any tips on how to fish because I've been fishing this area since 1949 and almost every year."*

I really thought I knew a lot about trout fishing and I do. However, I kept my mouth shut and my ears open. You can't learn with your mouth open. The long and the short of it is that we each caught our limit of trout that day using his method which was totally different than what we had done for years and years. Now, that's the only way that we fish and it has been proven to be far more successful than the way we fished before. To prove what I just said, we invited two friends to fish with us on a trip to Rock Creek Lake. All four rods and lines were rigged exactly the same way; our new way. We fished two days and all four of us caught our limits both days. We did not see anyone else along the shoreline catching fish the way we were and none of them had their limits.

So again I say it is a good idea to remain open minded even when you think you may know it all. You never know what you may learn. I like being an "open minded skeptic."

NONE ARE SO BLIND AS THOSE WHO REFUSE TO LOOK!

MY BELIEF SYSTEM INCLUDES, "THERE ARE NO INCURABLE ILLNESSES."

CHAPTER 10

LIST OF FAST FACTS

One major goal I have is to convince you that we have an enormous problem in our medical care system with the OVER-USE OF PRESCRIPTION DRUGS.

It should be noted that there are some drugs used for pain, surgery and other temporary situations which cannot be replaced or eliminated. They are critical to our well-being.

Now, when I look for a solution to a problem, I like to make sure I'm using logic. Here is what "old Benny" used to do when faced with a serious problem. You know the old Benny I mean; the guy with the long hair, funny square glasses and who was well-known for flying kites in the rain? Yes, that's right, old Ben Franklin. Old Benny was a highly intelligent man. He would make two lists on one piece of paper; one heading "Arguments in favor" and the other heading "Arguments opposed." Then he simply added up each column and the one with the longer list would be the winner. Let's try it.

Should we use prescription drugs for long-term treatment or try some other alternative or natural treatment?

* * *

Here are the arguments in favor of using prescription drugs:

Drugs are scientifically proven to be effective.
Drugs are simple to use—just take a pill.
Drugs act fast (and that's really good).
Most drugs do provide temporary relief to the health problem.

*   *   *

Here are the arguments opposed to using prescription drugs for long term treatment:

Pharmaceutical drugs do not treat the CAUSE and therefore DO NOT CURE (except for antibiotics).

Drugs are dangerous.

Believing in drugs is dangerous.

Drugs have NO HEALING PROPERTIES.

All prescription drugs are toxic.

Most drugs treat only the symptoms, but have no long-lasting benefit. They have temporary benefit only.

Prescription drugs kill—more drugs equal more deaths.

When a company spends more money on marketing than on producing their product, it usually means they have an inferior product.

We, in this country, have the shortest life span of all the developed countries in the world and we use more prescription drugs than any other country. It should be just the opposite if drugs were truly beneficial to us.

We are one of the sickest countries in the world with more chronically sick people than any other country and again we use more drugs. Before we became so addicted to drugs, we were in the top ten of the healthiest nations on earth.

All this evidence indicates that the benefits of drugs DO NOT outweigh the risks.

Most prescription drugs are very expensive.

There are natural treatments which can actually cure many illnesses.

*   *   *

OK folks, let's add them up. We now have four arguments in favor of and thirteen opposed.

Let me ask you, do you believe there is any question about the fact that prescription drugs are not always the best treatment?

*   *   *

Now that we've done that little exercise, let's review some more pertinent 'fast facts' about our medical system:

It costs General Motors over $1,500 per vehicle produced to provide health care insurance for their employees. It costs Toyota a little over $200 per vehicle.

The U.S.A. was in the top ten of the healthiest countries in the world, and now we are among the SICKEST COUNTRIES IN THE WHOLE WORLD.

We have a PROFIT-DRIVEN health care system. The focus is on profit, not cures.

In an interview on television, Mr. Kevin Trudeau made the statement that there is a law that says *"Only a drug can cure."*

If most drugs do not cure and doctors only prescribe drugs, then that means that most doctors are unable to CURE most illnesses.

Freedom of speech in medicine does not apply except for Big Pharma.

The drug companies have a POWERFUL INFLUENCE over the FDA.

The drug companies have a powerful influence over the FTC (Federal Trade Commission).

The drug used for chemotherapy for cancer has been the primary treatment recommended by your MD for over 50 years WITH NO SIGNIFICANT CHANGE.

Big Pharma promotes INDEPENDENT research that they pay for (if Big Pharma pays for the research, how can you call it independent?)

Big Pharma spends millions on lobbyists.

Big Pharma lobbyists outnumber senators five to one.

Big Pharma has the most elaborate and comprehensive marketing system ever.

The FDA has been suppressing all cancer cures and much more. For a real eye opener, just do a search on your computer for "FDA Suppression."

When people begin to die from a prescription drug, it appears that it takes a long time for the FDA to take any action.

Big Pharma has been caught bribing.

Big Pharma spends billions upon billions of dollars to SELL their products? Wouldn't you think that drugs should sell themselves, and all they would have to do is tell the doctors what their drugs do?

Big Pharma spends twice as much on promotion than they spend on research and development. TWICE AS MUCH ON PROMOTION AS ON RESEARCH. Did you hear an echo?

The TV audience is exposed to 16 hours a year of TV commercials about drug products.

The masses (that's us) are suckers for advertising whether it's true or not.

Big Pharma invents diseases for which they can provide a drug treatment.

The drug companies have convinced us that for them to make money is more important than our health.

It seems to me that there is a constant barrage of attorney advertisements on TV about class action lawsuits against the drug companies. It has been this way for several years now.

Drugs cannot be the only treatment available. Would God create a world that requires drugs only?

Drug companies can make more profit by developing a drug that only treats but does not cure, than if they developed a drug that would cure.

Students in med school are taught very little about nutrition.

There are medical scientists and there are medical doctors. The medical scientists know much more about the cause of illness than the medical doctors.

Medical scientists know the cause and cure for Parkinson's (for one example), but the medical doctors do not. There is one prescription drug and one pesticide that are known to cause Parkinson's.

The drug companies are scraping the bottom of the barrel to develop new drugs. They are developing new drugs to replace old drugs and some of the new ones are more dangerous and less effective.

They are also developing new drugs to PREVENT illness. Taking a toxic drug that could cause other illness, or even death, to prevent another illness, is ridiculous.

The former head of the Chinese FDA was executed for taking $850,000 in bribes from the drug companies. If that caught on here in the U.S., there could be a lot of dead people from all of the following: The FDA, AMA, FTC, NIH plus all of the universities that do clinical studies on food and drugs.

It is absolutely absurd for anyone to take any toxic substance for a long period of time, especially toxic prescription drugs. Drugs are fantastic for emergencies, surgeries, and other TEMPORARY situations.

The drug companies will make more money if they have a large and growing customer base.

During the last few decades, we are using more and more drugs and getting sicker and sicker. Could it be that the drugs are making us sicker?

The list of incurable illnesses is getting longer and not shorter.

Prescription drug use in the U.S.A. is higher than ever before and going higher.

Fifty-one percent of all children and adults are taking one or more drugs for a chronic condition.

Why do some drugs require a medical doctor's written prescription? Because they are DANGEROUS and they can kill people like you and me.

CHAPTER 11

MEDICAL DOCTORS

The first thing I want to say is most doctors I've met are "nice guys" and I'm sure most of them mean well. The problem is THE SYSTEM, and not the individual doctor. No doubt there are many good doctors who just don't fully realize the scope of the problem. They probably help many patients and are unaware of all the facts in this book. However, the biggest problem with our medical system involves prescription drugs and you can't buy them without a prescription from your medical doctor. Further, we learned in the Nazi war crime trials in Nuremberg, Germany, that following orders does not excuse us from responsibility.

One more thing about doctors before I say another word:

THE DOCTOR DID NOT CAUSE YOUR ILLNESS; YOU DID. Most of our illnesses are self-inflicted.

We, that means you and I, are the cause of most of our illnesses by our negligence in the care and maintenance of our bodies. And then, when we eventually have a health problem, we run to the MD and that's where our problems begin to get worse.

This is a short story about TRUST. We trust our medical doctors, so let's talk about trust.

I worked most of my adult life for a large insurance company and in a variety of jobs. For about three years, my job as an underwriter was to review all business insurance claims for most of Southern California after they were paid. One of the many coverages provided by a business insurance policy is Employee Dishonesty. Based on my review of many, many claims for this coverage, it was determined that the employee who most often stole money or property from their employer was the trusted bookkeeper or the head accountant. Also, these claims were for large amounts of money. Now, here's where the trust comes in. In almost every situation, the bookkeeper or accountant was the most TRUSTED employee. My conclusion is that you cannot trust any one person with a large amount of property or money for a long period of time. The temptation is just too great. There may be exceptions, but how do you know?

Medical doctors are among the most trusted people on earth. Many of us TRUST them with our lives, and I mean it literally.

Over a period of time, too much trust will lead to an unpleasant end and that is just what is happening.

The number of people you can trust reduces as the dollar amount increases and the length of time the temptation exists.

The following story is an example of why you cannot trust ALL doctors. There is a TV series called "AMERICAN GREED." In January 2009, they had a true story about a skin doctor in Florida. The doctor was telling almost every patient who had a skin biopsy that it was cancerous. Additionally, he almost always did a four-layer surgery, which is the maximum. The removal of each layer of skin is a separate surgery. Normally, one or two layers is all that is needed. Obviously, the doctor was doing everything to maximize his profit. Here is where the trust comes in. When the investigators interviewed the patients, it was quite apparent that they trusted him completely, because none of them ever considered a second opinion. The problem is too much trust creates too much temptation.

This doctor is now serving 22 years in the penitentiary.

Let's talk about doctors now and the role they play in our medical system. A doctor must be a fairly intelligent person to be accepted into a medical school. He or she probably comes from a fairly well-to-do family who can afford the cost. They probably know very little about health care in the beginning. Therefore, they do not question what they are being taught. So they can be molded anyway desired. They learn a lot about the body and a lot about prescription drugs and some basics about surgery. BUT, I about fell out of my chair when I learned that they are taught almost nothing about nutrition. After all, why teach them something they may never use. Nutrition is in direct conflict with the sale of prescription drugs.

OK, let's say you graduate from medical school and open your office. It will probably take you some time, maybe even a few years, to realize that you are not curing anyone. You may wonder why you ever got into this, but down deep you know. Surveys of medical students have repeatedly shown that 90% want to be a doctor FOR THE MONEY. So what do you do now? You've spent all this money and time in medical school and treating patients to realize this. Well, doctors just don't change careers at this point. You either continue doing what you're doing and/or you write a book about what you've learned. Time for a reminder: I'm alive today only because of the Internet and those doctors who write books. I thank them again.

One thing they do that I really don't like is argue with the patient when the patient tells them about their problem. I've had that experience when I told the doctor something, and he replied *"That can't be."*

Here is an example right out of the newspaper: The "Los Angeles Times" has a once-a-week Health Section where they post letters from their readers and answer their questions. Recently, a lady wrote that she was taking several prescription drugs and developed pain, weakness and eventually could not walk. The lady looked up her medications to determine possible drug interaction and she found one. She told her doctor about it and he said *"There is no interaction."* Now, how do you like that for an answer? The lady stopped one of the two drugs and within four weeks she had dramatic improvement. About two months later, she saw her doctor again and because her cholesterol was high, he ordered another drug. Now I ask you, how important is it for an 86 year old woman with no history of heart disease, to lower her cholesterol. I just don't get it. It is not logical. I think her doctor is dangerous.

Here's another letter from an 81 year old woman. She writes that she is taking amitriptyline, Aricept, Arthrotec, aspirin, Avapro, Chlor-Trimeton, Levothroid, Lexapro, Lortab, Norvase, Symbicort and Tylenol Arthritis. She complains that she's dizzy all the time and it's getting worse. She wants to know if the drugs may be the cause. Well you and I both know the answer to that.

I really question the use of antidepressant drugs. I don't think the doctors are using their noggins when you consider just some of the side effects, which include insomnia, teeth grinding at night, sweating, muscle spasms, nightmares, constant fatigue, headaches, nausea, diarrhea, and hair loss.

These kinds of medical doctors mentioned in the three previous stories, in my opinion, are no better than LICENSED drug salesmen.

Here is what I think about doctors prescribing drugs. When they write a prescription, they should be telling the patient this: *"Take these pills everyday and I assure you they will only treat your symptoms and never cure you. Also, they are toxic (that means poison) and have awful side effects and possibly even death."* Now, can't you and I just imagine them doing that? Ha-ha-ha!

There are hundreds of studies that prove alternative treatments are effective for many health problems. Why do doctors ignore all that and only prescribe drugs.

Hippocrates is known as the "Father of Medicine" and he said *"Let food be your medicine and medicine be your food."* Why do the doctors of today ignore that? Was Hippocrates wrong? I don't think so.

Here are a couple of stories that are good examples of what I like least about MD's. I told you the story about my experience with one doctor and the drug Flagyl. After I had been taking Flagyl three times without any success, I went to Orange County Health Department and the doctor there told me how to take Flagyl and Odoxin. When I went back to my doctor and told him what I wanted to do, he said *"It won't make any difference."* That response tells me that his ego is super large and he is a know-it-all and further, he did not want to learn from his patients. He never did learn because I never went back to him to tell him of my success.

This story is about a different doctor who did my prostate surgery that I call the "roto-rooter" surgery. As a result of the surgery, one part of my anatomy was one and a half inches shorter than before. When I told the doctor about it, he said "That can't be." Well, that shocked me and irritated the hell out of me; he just did not give a damn and he might as well have accused me of lying. I did not like his whole attitude and I never saw him again.

The book about my ALS successful experience was first published about four to five years ago. Along with that, we established a web site. From these two endeavors, we began to get a lot of e-mail from our readers who are mostly PALS (Person with ALS); about five or ten e-mail a day for over four years. That's well over 1,000 a year. So it is no exaggeration that we have been in communication with literally thousands of PALS. Almost without exception, they all tell the same exact story, about what their medical doctors told them. They were all told that there is no cure or treatment and they should go home and put their affairs in order. They also tell PALS *"Don't even look for cures, because there aren't any."* I believe that's not true and could be a BIG LIE. Now, if I were a doctor in that situation, I would be inclined to tell my patient that I could do nothing. However, you might want to consult with other health care professionals. BUT, doctors don't do that. I wonder why? It seems to me that they have all been coached to say exactly the same thing.

Let me remind you that I have successfully treated my ALS condition and some would consider that miraculous. So, I'm either a miracle man or most all of our doctors are stupid. I mean, what other explanation is there? Well, I'm no miracle man and I don't believe our doctors are really stupid. There is one other possibility and that could only be the way they are taught in med school. What do you think? Is there any other explanation that you can think of? I don't think so.

There is one indication that doctors may be limited in their choice of treatments. It seems to me that they avoid any and all anecdotal stories like mine where someone has developed a cure for an illness. They simply do not want to know about it. The entire medical community ignores all anecdotal evidence like it's beneath them and it's not scientific. Well let me ask you this: How did we learn that toad stools were poison and mushrooms were OK? I believe the evidence was all anecdotal.

Our doctors not only claim there is no cure, but they also claim that they do not know the cause or even have a clue. In my opinion, what they really mean to say is that they do not have a drug for ALS. There is one drug, Rilutek, but it simply does not work and most doctors never prescribe it.

Now let me tell you how wrong that is and explain how utterly simple the real truth is. ALS is a NEURO degenerative illness. I emphasize neuro because the problem is centered in your nervous system. Also there are many toxins which are labeled NEURO toxins. They are called neuro because these toxins attack the nervous system. It is well known that neuro toxins cause muscle atrophy and weakness. It is also well known that the primary symptoms of ALS are exactly the same.

There are many neuro toxins, but probably the number one toxin causing ALS is Mercury. The only question about whether or not it could be a cause of ALS is whether or not you are exposed to it in any volume. Now, let me tell you. We voluntarily put Mercury in our teeth (more on that later). It is a well-known fact that most fish you buy in the market or that you catch contain Mercury well beyond a safe level. Mercury has also been used in shots and vaccinations for years. Mercury is also one of many toxins that are put into our atmosphere by coal burning power plants and other industrial factories.

There is absolutely no doubt about Mercury being a significant toxin and there is absolutely no doubt that we are exposed to it in volume. Also, there is no safe limit for Mercury in your body. Even the smallest amount can and will eventually cause you a health problem. One more thing, there is absolutely no doubt that most medical doctors do not know much about Mercury and they have no test to diagnose the amount of any heavy metal in your body. They do test your blood, but a blood test only tells you if you have massive amounts of heavy metals in your body. It does not tell you what's in your body tissue, and that's where the heavy metals and other toxins are stored. Doctors also use a urine test, but that only tells you what toxins are being eliminated, not what's in there. There is a test called a hair analysis, but most doctors simply don't believe in it. Maybe they are not taught to believe in it.

When medical examiners are performing autopsies and they have reason to suspect poison, they use a hair analysis. Why don't doctors use it? So, medical examiners use a hair analysis to determine the cause of death, but medical doctors DO NOT use a hair analysis to determine a cause of illness. Does that make sense to you? I don't think so.

There is more than one drug company doing research to develop a drug for ALS. Part of their research involves testing on mice. Question: Where do they find mice with ALS? Answer: They don't find them, they must create them. How? I've been told that they inject them with Mercury to give them ALS. How about that sports fans?

It appears to me that Dr. Benjamin Rush was absolutely right in his prediction way back in 1776. He predicted that medicine would organize into an undercover dictatorship. They could then limit both competition and new medical advances. It looks to me as though that is exactly what is happening now.

What are you supposed to do when your doctor tells you no cure is available and go home and die? Should you just give up and die? I don't think so. I know there are cures. Since your doctor admits he cannot help you, then the only choice is to divorce him and seek help from other health care professionals.

Thousands of us will die every year from environmental toxins such as Arsenic, Mercury, and on and on. Does your doctor know how to treat or prevent this from occurring? I don't think so.

A clever way to murder your spouse is by administering small doses of Arsenic over a long period of time. The patient will get sick and go to the doctor but the doctor will rarely diagnose it correctly. Heavy metals like Arsenic and Mercury stay in the body and accumulate eventually causing death. I have seen three different TV documentaries where one spouse has killed the other spouse by this method. In one story, the killer did not get caught until after she murdered her eleventh husband.

Lesson: Doctors do not appear to know much about poison or toxins.

Another thing about most medical doctors is the wait. You have an APPOINTMENT, but you still wait up to one or two hours for a five minute appointment. That really annoys me. I think my time is just as valuable to me as theirs is to them.

Here is one of my biggest complaints. I truly believe that MD's have a moral and ethical obligation to tell you about not only the dangers of prescription drugs, but also that they probably WILL NOT CURE. I have never had a doctor tell me that the drug he was prescribing would not provide a cure. Also, I've only had one doctor in over 50 years tell me about the horrible side effects of any drug.

Several years ago I read an article about doctors and minor surgery. There is a greater frequency of tonsillectomies in areas with poorer economies. Evidently, the doctors need more money so any borderline situation goes right to the hospital.

In a more recent article written by an MD, it was believed that hysterectomies and caesarian births were only necessary about half of the time. Again, the economic factor enters the picture. Remember my gallbladder story earlier in the book? Same thing.

Although many medical doctors will deny that the drug companies influence them with the many billions of dollars they spend on them, there are indications that most doctors favor the drug companies. Here is a story that might convince you of this:

A person wrote into the "Los Angeles Times" and her letter was published March 2, 2009. The person said they had been taking Synthroid and Levoxyl for over 15 years. Those are both prescription drugs for thyroid. They went on to say that their medical doctor wanted to reduce the dose because the doctor was worried about it might weaken their bones. The person listed many problem symptoms that they thought were related to the reduced thyroid. Now, I'm not a doctor, but my common sense tells me that that's not very bright. You might remember that in an earlier chapter I wrote about my thyroid problem. I have been taking a NATURAL thyroid hormone called Armour thyroid for about 50 years and no problems. If the doctor was REALLY concerned about the patient's bone density, then he should have prescribed NATURAL thyroid like I take. Armour is not a drug so there are no bad side effects that I know about. The way I see this, and I may be wrong, is that the MD has a moral and ethical obligation to tell his patient of any and all options. In this case, the option is a drug or a natural hormone. I'm certain that the natural hormone would be preferred by the patient. Maybe the doctor doesn't know about Armour thyroid. Well, in my opinion, whether he does or does not, what he is doing is irresponsible. Maintaining a proper dose of thyroid is absolutely critical to good health. I don't know about you, but this kind of thing makes me mad, but I don't know whether to be mad at the doctor or the drug companies. I only hope and believe that all doctors are not like this one, but it is a good example.

I do not enjoy saying this, but the following information was taken from a web site and based on a report in the "<u>New York Times</u>." The crux of the story is that many doctors are abusive and arrogant and that their attitude leads to mistakes and even fatalities. I have met many doctors in my lifetime that I felt were arrogant and egocentric. I think that medical school teaches them to be that way. Medical doctors THINK their way is the ONLY way, but they are dead wrong.

Profile of a Good Doctor—My Doctor

Now for a breath of fresh air and sunshine about medical doctors. I have a good one, but they are as rare as "hen's teeth." There are some good doctors like mine and I would like to tell you why I think they are good and what a good doctor should be.

The story about my good doctor begins prior to my first visit. Because of my ALS condition, I could not talk very well when I first went to him. So, I brought a message to be read to him by my wife. It went something like this:

"I'm looking for a good doctor to help me with my ALS condition. I want a person with medical knowledge to provide me with counsel and advice. I'm looking for a partner, and not one who will dictate to me. I would like to know all of my options and in the final analysis, I will make the decisions about any treatment. Will you accept me as your patient based on that?"

Fortunately for me, he accepted me as a patient. I have had many really good experiences with Dr. Neal Rouzier of Palm Springs, California over the last 13 years. Some things he has recommended I have done and some I have not. However, we get along famously and that's the way it should be. I have recommended him to many others and continue to do so. One really good example is that he LISTENS to me, and I listen to him. He seems never to be in a hurry to be done with me. Many of his recommendations have helped in my improvement.

In spite of all that I've said about doctors, there may be hope yet. What we really need are doctors who are trained not only in drugs but also alternative treatments. There are a few doctors doing that right now.

Locate an ACAM (American College for Advancement in Medicine) Doctor

ACAM is a not-for-profit medical society. Most of these doctors do Chelation and other alternative treatments. However, not all of them have the same degree of Chelation training. You still must be selective in your choice of a doctor.

ACAM represents more than 1,000 physicians in many countries. To find one in your area, you can contact them at the address below or look on their web site:

The American College for Advancement in Medicine
23121 Verdugo Dr., Suite 204
Laguna Hills, CA 92653
Phone (949) 583-7666 or Toll Free Outside CA (800) 532-3688
http://www.acam.org/

There are other examples of what I call really good doctors. They are the ones who learn about real cures. These maverick doctors, who are responsible for saving my life, have written many books trying to blow the whistle on the present system. The problem is, however, very few people read the books, but I read them. Here is just one example: The title is "Detoxify or Die" written by Sherry Rogers, MD. Now, get this folks. Here is a doctor telling us to detoxify or we will die, and yet our medical system has no approved treatment to detoxify. Here is a doctor who is really trying to help us. There is another book titled "Alkalize or Die" by Dr. Theodore A. Baroody. The title of these two books should raise your interest. Here are two medical doctors writing about two different life-threatening situations that the average MD knows nothing about.

There are two forms of IV Chelation that can be very beneficial to our health, and yet most medical doctors don't use them. It may be just the way they are taught. One is for treating Lead poisoning known as EDTA. The other is DMPS which is for treating Mercury poisoning. It is my understanding that the only time doctors use either of these is when the Mercury or Lead shows up in a blood or urine test. The problem is that these and other heavy metals don't always show up in a blood or urine test because they are stored in the body tissue. They will show up in a hair analysis, but that's another test that most MD's do not use. I believe, from my own experience, that a small amount of heavy metal toxicity can cause many illnesses such as ALS. One of my major treatments to save my life from ALS was the IV Chelation with DMPS to remove Mercury. I find it difficult to understand why our MD's don't know about this and don't use Chelation to treat illness.

My Summation

The main purpose of this chapter is to show you how to live with them by using your MD only for diagnosis, emergencies, physical traumas and other life-threatening situations. If you are sick and no emergency, then you may have a better chance of surviving by seeking some other type of health care professional and/or reading a lot of books like I did or find an MD who will answer "Yes" to most of the questions in the following quiz:

We receive over 1000 e-mail every year from ALS patients who have read my book "Eric is Winning" and have questions. I received an e-mail the other day that began this way: "I went to two doctors and they have told me to forget the natural way. I was so upset." That really bothers me because I hear all the time that doctors tell their patients, as they did me, to avoid alternative treatments. I have a difficulty understanding why they do that and I believe they should not do that. If they have any personal experience, personal knowledge, or detailed information about any specific alternative treatment that has proven to be ineffective, then fine, tell their patient that. BUT to tell their patients that ALL alternative treatments are ineffective is very, very wrong in my opinion. THERE IS NO WAY THAT ANY ONE DOCTOR CAN POSSIBLY KNOW THAT MUCH ABOUT ALL HEALTH CARE TREATMENTS IN THE WHOLE WORLD. That defies logic.

This e-mail caused me to really think about this problem and I have developed a quiz for medical doctors. I would really like to know how most MD's would answer these questions. Also, if I ever am looking for a new MD, I would ask them to take this quiz before I would accept them as my doctor. You might consider doing the same thing. At least it would be an eye-opener.

* * *

QUIZ FOR YOUR MD

Do you believe that some alternative treatments are effective?
Do you ever recommend alternative treatments for your patients?

Do you believe that prescription drugs are not the only treatment for illnesses?

Do you believe that nutrition has a role in health care?

Do you believe that nutrition has a role in the prevention of illness?

Do you believe that nutrition can be effective in the treatment of illness?

Thousands of us die every year from air pollution. Do you understand that toxins are the real cause of these deaths?

Do you understand that toxins are also in most of our food and water?

Since most people get very sick before they die, do you have any tests which will indicate that your patient may die from toxic pollution?

Do you regularly test your patients for nutritional deficiency which may be the cause of their illness?

Do you know that Mercury is toxic?

Do you believe toxic Mercury should never be used for dental fillings?

Do you understand that MSG and Aspartame are both highly toxic and are the cause of much illness?

Do you believe in treating the CAUSE of your patient's illness?

Do you know that most prescription drugs rarely cure any illness other than antibiotics?

Since most statin drugs have proven to be ineffective in preventing heart attacks, have you ceased prescribing them?

Do you ever refer your patients to a chiropractor?

Do you know that IV Chelation with EDTA can prevent heart attacks?

Dr. Ignarro was awarded a Nobel Prize in Medicine in 1998 for his discovery that nitric oxide can prevent many illnesses including heart disease. Have you included this in your treatment program that you recommend to your patients?

Do you tell your patients that cancer thrives on sugar, thrives in an acidic and low oxygen environment, and that Vitamin D (sunshine) helps prevent cancer?

NOTE: If I were looking for a medical doctor, I would love to find one who could answer "Yes" to all of the these questions.

*   *   *

The long and the short of it is this. You should not put too much trust in any doctor. You and you alone are responsible for your health. You cannot delegate that RESPONSIBILITY. Before having any surgery or taking any drug LONG TERM, I strongly recommend that you obtain a second or even a third opinion. You should be an open-minded skeptic like me, and be skeptical of any doctor who ONLY recommends drugs or surgery. This could lengthen your life by many years.

The number of gun owners in this country is 80 million. The number of accidental gun deaths per year, all age groups, is about 1500. The number of accidental deaths per gun owner is 0.000188.

The number of medical doctors in the U.S. is about 700,000. The number of accidental deaths caused by doctors per year is 120,000 (that is a bare minimum). The number of accidental deaths per doctor is 0.171.

The result of this comparison is that doctors are 9,000 times more dangerous than gun owners. Should we really ban guns? Or, are we banning the wrong enemy?

When I was first married way back in 1950, my father-in-law gave me some of the best advice ever, but I did not realize how good it was until now. He said *"Avoid lawyers and medical doctors.*

CHAPTER 12

THE COUP DE GRACE

This is my last shot at our medical care system.

I have never ever seen a complete compilation of the number of deaths caused by the ENTIRE MEDICAL CARE SYSTEM.UNTIL NOW.

These figures may differ considerably from the figures I told you about earlier in this book because they were based on drugs only. I want to emphasize that all previous numbers of sickness and death were all related to only prescription drugs. No one, to my knowledge, had ever combined all the statistical evidence in one shocking report on not only drugs but the entire medical system. So, you better sit down and have the smelling salts handy. The following information was taken from an article "Death by Medicine" found on the Life Extension web site. Credit for the article goes to three medical doctors and two PhD's: Gary Null, PhD; Carolyn Dean MD, ND; Martin Feldman, MD; Debora Rasio, MD; and Dorothy Smith, PhD.

Now are you ready? Here we go.

The number of UNNECESSARY medical and SURGICAL procedures performed annually is 7.5 million per year.

The number of people UNNECESSARILY HOSPITALIZED annually is 8.9 million per year.

When a drug company FUNDS a study, there is a 90% chance that the drug will be perceived as effective but when a NON-DRUG COMPANY PAYS for the study, it will show favorable results only 50% of the time.

U.S. health care spending reached $1.6 trillion in 2003. That is 14% of our gross national product.

It is estimated that under-reporting of medical errors amounts to 5% to 20% of the actual number of occurrences.

It is also estimated that only 6% of adverse drug events are identified properly.

One out of four patients suffers observable side effects from prescription drugs.

In 2002, there were more than 3.34 billion prescriptions for drugs filled.

That is 12 prescriptions for every living person in the U.S.A. Now you know that babies and children are not getting that many and there are 40 million uninsured who are probably not getting their share either. That means that many, many people must be getting 15 or 20 EVERY YEAR.

One study indicates that over half of the new drugs develop serious post-approval risks.

Every year there are over 3 million pounds of antibiotics used by human beings.

Almost all respiratory infections are VIRAL and antibiotics are not effective on them, but they use them anyway. Isn't that kind of dumb?

German biostatistician, Ulrich Abel, PhD, wrote a paper on chemotherapy. He concluded that there is no direct evidence that chemotherapy prolongs survival in patients with advanced cancers.

There are about 2.4 million UNNECESSARY SURGERIES performed in one year (1974).

These unnecessary surgeries resulted in 11,900 deaths in that same year.

In 2001, the number of unnecessary surgeries was up to 7.5 million (up more than 300%).

In that same year, there were 37,136 deaths resulting from those unnecessary surgeries.

I don't know about you folks, but my reaction is this: THAT IS UNACCEPTABLE.

It is estimated that x-rays, CT scans, mammography and fluoroscopy devices are a major contributing factor in new cancers. Birth control pills also contribute.

In 2001, there were about 4 million births in the U.S.A. and 24% were by cesarean. In the Netherlands, cesarean section represents only 8% of their births. I imagine that doctors make more money performing cesarean sections.

AND NOW FOLKS WE HAVE WHAT YOU'VE BEEN WAITING FOR. THE BOTTOM LINE.

The two leading causes of death in the U.S.A. are THOUGHT to be cancer and heart disease. In 2001, there were just under 700,000 heart disease deaths and about 550,000 cancer deaths.

NOW FOR THE SHOCKING NEWS. IN THE SAME YEAR, THERE WERE JUST UNDER 800,000 DEATHS CAUSED BY CONVENTIONAL MEDICINE.

Assuming these figures are correct, that means that our highly regarded medical system is really THE NUMBER ONE KILLER OF PEOPLE IN THE U.S.A.

But wait a minute, we said earlier that only 5% to 20% of medical errors were ever reported. If that holds true here, then the figure of 800,000 is probably way too low. The fact is we don't know. BUT, if those percentages apply, then the FDA, Big Pharma and MD's could be responsible for about five times that amount or 4 million. Golly, what do you make of that? Our medical system could really be responsible for 4 million deaths every year? That is a BEHEMOTH of a number.

Boy oh boy, didn't that just blow your barn doors off at the hinges? Some of those figures should have shaken you right down to your foundation.

Whatever happened to that part of the Hippocratic Oath that says something like this:

"FIRST, DO NO HARM."

With all of these death statistics, you might be wondering this.

The definition of manslaughter is *"The unlawful killing of a human being without express or implied malice."*

The medical system in this country is like a big machine—a massive relentless machine crushing whatever lies in its path leaving hundreds of thousands dead in its wake—a true juggernaut with no single entity at the controls.

Where is the caped crusader when you really need him?

Remember, this was predicted by Dr. Benjamin Rush. Imagine that, a medical doctor and a signer of the U.S. Constitution knew in advance that this might happen if we did not include a provision for FREEDOM OF MEDICINE.

CHAPTER 13

PREVENTION
PART ONE—INTRODUCTION

Up to this point, this book has been filled with negative information about health care. NOW, we will switch to more positive "stuff." The next few chapters are all about what can help you live a longer and better life.

Although there are some contrarians who believe we cannot do anything to help us live longer, I think they are full of "hops." I KNOW WE CAN LIVE LONGER if we know and do just some of the things in the next two chapters. To prove what I just said, we know that the Seventh-day Adventists live to an average age of 88, and that's about 10 years longer than normal. That may be due to their non-smoking, their diet and their involvement with family and religion. I believe they eat more vegetables and more of it organic.

It might help you to know why I believe I have been healthy most of my life before ALS. First of all, I think my mother was one of the brightest mothers in the whole world. The way she raised me and taught me was almost ideal and very different from the way kids are raised today. Here are some of the particulars:

My mother fed me on breast milk for the first few months of my life. She never used any canned milk or baby's milk formula. I really think that is a great way to start your life. Then, she fed me table food only. I ate whatever the adults ate. All you have to do is mash up the food with a fork to make it more suitable for a baby. As a result, my mother told me I NEVER threw up. That went on for a long time and the first time I ever threw up in my whole life was when I drank too much alcohol when I was about 16.

My mother had a lot of fresh fruit available for me. We NEVER had candy, coke or cookies in our home. A candy bar or a soft drink was a RARE treat.

We never had a sugar bowl on the table. I learned to eat cold cereal and/or oatmeal without any sugar.

All through my young life, I left the house in the early morning and headed to school or went out to play. I NEVER remained in the house watching TV or listening to the radio. I would stay out all day until the street lights came on and that's when my mother expected me home and I never disappointed her. When I was outside, I was always physically active in some sport. Exercise, fresh air and sunshine are, I believe, very important to a growing child.

Here's one last item that is very important. I love vegetables and fresh fruit. I learned that from my mother. Here's how she did it. My mother would dish up a moderate helping of every food on the table. I had to eat everything on my plate if I wanted seconds on anything else. That's how I learned to like almost all foods. I would eat almost anything to get more fresh beets. I loved them. We rarely had dessert, but if we did, I also had to eat everything on my plate first.

Now, that's my background. I am 79 years old and healthier than most people my age minus the ALS and I believe I owe it to my mother and the way I was raised. I am probably the healthiest man with ALS that you'll ever hear about.

The next chapter will tell you about more things you might want to KNOW to prevent and/or treat illness and then later there will be another chapter about things to DO to prevent and/or treat illness.

CHAPTER 14

PREVENTION
PART TWO—THINGS TO KNOW

Before we begin, we should review some facts about the cause of health problems and remind you about who I am. I am not a health care professional. Also, everything in here is based on my own personal experience and/or books and articles written by health care professionals. Remember, I had to learn all this in order to begin treating my so-called incurable disease—ALS (Lou Gehrig's disease). I am a living test laboratory. Because of my ALS condition, I am highly susceptible to anything toxic AND I am also highly reactive to any good food or supplement. I am fairly sure of what I say in this chapter, but remember that I am not a doctor.

Most of what I have learned about health care I have read somewhere and then confirmed it with my own experiences. Many others write about their opinion or their theory. I'm one of the few people who write about my actual results from eating certain foods or taking certain supplements; my writing is based primarily on that and not on theory alone.

You might need to know that we mention no BRAND NAMES of any product. To do that may bring down the wrath of the "Medical Mafia."

One more thing, you must know that you are in control and no one else. You have the ability to not smoke, lose weight, or follow any diet that YOU WANT TO. So, don't think that you can't do this or that. My grandmother used to say *"There's no such word as can't."*

Remember, there are only two reasons why you don't do something: you are physically incapable or you simply don't want to. So, never confuse can't with won't.

There are three things of utmost importance that you must know. One is that drugs do not cure (with rare exceptions), and the second is most medical doctors use only drugs to treat illness. Thirdly, you should understand what causes illness and treat the cause.

TO KNOW THE CAUSE IS TO KNOW THE CURE. You must know the cause of the problem in order to correct or successfully treat the problem.

You must know that there are no incurable illnesses. There is a possible cure for everything if you search for it. In fact, there's a book written by a medical doctor titled "There Are No Incurable Diseases" by Dr. Richard Schulze. See his web site for more information:

http://www.herbdoc.com/home_1024x768.asp

Now don't miss this. Here we have a MEDICAL DOCTOR who is stating clearly that there are no incurable illnesses. That's the exact opposite of what most other MD's tell us. I wonder who is telling the truth?

Here is another book you might read written by a DOCTOR. The author says many of the same things I say in this book. The title of the book is "The Cure—The 12-Week Plan to Prevent and Reverse Cancer, Heart Disease, Obesity and More" by Dr. Timothy Brantley.

If you are looking for a CURE and not just temporary relief, then you must seek and find other treatments—I really mean you should look to "Mother Nature." SHE does not use drugs and she has been around a lot longer than drugs.

PERHAPS AS MUCH AS 80% OF ALL ILLNESS IS CAUSED BY NUTRITIONAL DEFICIENCY AND/OR ENVIRONMENTAL TOXINS.

There is one notable exception to the above statement. MISALIGNMENT OF THE SPINAL COLUMN CAN CAUSE SERIOUS ILLNESS AND IS BEST TREATED BY A CHIROPRACTOR. Their modern techniques produce amazing results.

Most of the remaining 20% of our illnesses are caused by infectious diseases resulting from pathogens such as bacteria, viruses, fungi, protozoa, protein, mycoplasmas and other parasites. It is estimated that over 60 million people in the U.S.A. are likely infected with a parasite associated with RAW meat and contact with cat feces. Another 50 million children are infected with worm parasites. Now, folks, that's only two of the many, many pathogens we are exposed to everyday. I believe that all of us probably have one or more pathogens in our bodies.

The Basics of Healing

The father of medicine, Hippocrates, said *"Let your food be your medicine and your medicine be your food."*

If you eat no food, you will get sick and die in about 30 days. If you eat only plastic and cardboard, you will have the same result. You must have NUTRIENT-RICH food to be healthy. You cannot just eat anything you want.

You may also die prematurely from our toxin-polluted environment.

If you desire a long life and/or a healthy life, you must have PURE water, a variety of nutritional and NON-TOXIC foods, and CLEAN air. Thousands of us die every year from pollution (see Death by Pollution below). Toxins are in our air, water and food. The government does very little to correct this problem and most medical doctors are not interested in prevention. The drug companies love it; the more sick people, the more customers for them. We must get back to a more natural life; more natural foods, more exercise and avoid toxins.

Wild animals live in an ALL NATURAL world with nothing artificial. They eat raw, fresh and unmodified foods. They drink pure water. They are outdoors 24/7 with plenty of sunshine. Oh yes, they all get a lot of exercise.

"Well, Eric, so what? We like our way of life."

We all like the way we live, but this artificial world shortens our lives. Wild animals have a life expectancy of 2 to 1 to ours. That is, if one does not eat the other. They do this without any medical doctors and without any prescription drugs. 'Golly gee,' imagine that! They outlive us, without any drugs. When you stop and think about it, that's pretty amazing. By the way, most mammals live to be seven times their age at maturity. Assuming we mature at age 20, then we should live to be 140.

If you read the obituaries, you will realize that almost no one dies of natural causes and we are all dying prematurely. That is not natural, so let me tell you how it should be in a short story.

One of my best friends had an uncle who lived in Texas. When the uncle was in his 90's, a cowboy magazine wrote an article about him because he was the oldest living, working cowboy in the U.S. He died a few years later, but how he died is the whole story. When he did not return to the ranch house one day, they went out looking for him. They found him laying down on his back on the ground with the reins to his horse in his hands. It appeared as though he got off his horse and laid down to rest or take a nap. Now, that folks is the way it is supposed to happen.

No medical doctor or anyone else in the entire world can heal you or me of anything. ALL HEALING OCCURS WITHIN THE BODY AND BY THE BODY. All anyone can do is to be an assistant to that process. From the date of conception, the body grows and develops based entirely on the nutrients it receives. Our health continues only as long as the nutrients are there. We must have the nutrients in fresh, high quality food to sustain life. Our bodies do not require drugs to live a healthy life. Several decades ago, medical doctors relied on special diets to actually cure illness. Today, that is long gone.

THE DOCTORS OF TODAY WILL BECOME THE NUTRITIONISTS OF TOMORROW, OR THE NUTRITIONISTS OF TODAY WILL BECOME THE DOCTORS OF TOMORROW.

When the body becomes overwhelmed with too many toxins for it to handle or eliminate, the body stores the toxins in the body tissue and organs. This leads to eventual illness and/or death. The obvious solution is to help the body eliminate the toxins. To my knowledge, our MD's have no approved treatment to do this.

There is a lot more you need to know about what causes illness. You especially need to know about POLLUTION, AMALGAM DENTAL FILLINGS, MSG (Monosodium Glutamate), ASPARTAME and the MIRACLE OF pH.

Now for a discussion of each one of those:

Death by Pollution

The following information was taken from an article in the "Los Angeles Times" May 22, 2008:

24,000 deaths annually in California are linked to chronic exposure to fine particulate pollution of the air.

These figures are based on new research across the nation about the hazards posed by microscopic particles which sink deep into the lungs. This included several major studies occurring over the last five years. The studies found that the rate of heart attacks, strokes and other serious disease increased exponentially after exposure to even slightly higher amounts of metal, dust or other fragments from tail pipes and smoke stacks.

There's no death certificate that says specifically someone died of air pollution, but cities with higher rates of air pollution have much greater rates of death from cardiovascular diseases. Californians exposed to high levels of particulates had their lives cut short by an average of 10 years. Researchers also found that when particulates are cut even temporarily, death rates fall.

When Dublin imposed a coal ban, when Hong Kong imposed reductions in sulfur dioxide, when there was a steel mill strike in Utah, they all saw immediate reductions in deaths.

The economic cost attributed to premature deaths in California alone is estimated to be $70 billion annually.

Another article in the "Los Angeles Times" on 9-30-08 discussed the new California state regulation about toxins in certain products. California launched a very comprehensive program to regulate toxic chemicals which have been linked to cancer and other deadly illnesses. These new laws are designed to regulate 80,000 chemicals which are now in use. That's right, folks, 80,000. I mention this figure just to give you an idea of how polluted our world is; polluted with toxins that cause you and I health problems.

These articles from the "Los Angeles Times" CONVINCE ME that the theory about toxins and death is real. This information proves to me that cholesterol is not the cause of heart attacks and other illnesses. Rather, this is further evidence that TOXINS are one of the main causes of illness.

Water Pollution

Most tap water in this country contains chlorine. Chlorine is a known toxin and a known carcinogen. We need something to purify the water but it should not be toxic. If we must use a toxin like chlorine, then we should at least warn the public. Most people don't know that. The main reason why people are buying bottled water to drink is to avoid chlorine. I've had many outdoor koi fish ponds and three times after cleaning out the pond and putting in fresh tap water, all my koi fish died. That should give you an idea of just how dangerous tap water is when it contains chlorine.

Amalgam Dental Fillings

What they call amalgam dental fillings, you may know as Silver fillings. However, amalgam fillings contain more Mercury than Silver. Mercury is highly toxic and more toxic than Arsenic. It is second only to Uranium. Mercury is the number one NEURO toxin. Mercury has the ability to penetrate the blood/brain barrier and damage the motor neurons. When any neuro toxin, especially Mercury, damages the motor neurons, you will have muscle atrophy and weakness.

The American Dental Association would have us believe that this hazardous material is only hazardous before and after, but when it's in your mouth, it is perfectly safe. If you believe that, I would like to sell you some ocean front property in Arizona.

The Federal government does not want old amalgam dental fillings to wind up in our landfills for obvious reasons; they are poison. And yet the Federal government does not warn us about the hazards of the exact same material being in your mouth. Does that make sense? I don't think so.

Sometime way back in the 1840s, dentists began using amalgam dental fillings. However, the Dental Association was opposed to the use of amalgams (and for a good reason). The dentists objected and formed a new Dental Association that would approve of their use of amalgams. Who knows how many thousands of people have suffered and died from that simple decision? It was only a few years later in the 1860's when we had the first ALS diagnosis.

Isn't that a strange coincidence?

Mercury is poison and does not belong in your mouth.

I've read many stories about people who have suffered with many illnesses, then removed their amalgam fillings and recovered their health. That's why they are eliminating Mercury from thermometers, thermostats, and much more.

There are many people fighting to abolish the use of amalgam dental fillings and they have been doing it for many years. You may not be aware of it, but they are. There have been many lawsuits regarding amalgams, and some have been in our favor. About one year ago a dentist lost a suit against the makers of amalgams, BUT the court did agree on one thing. AMALGAMS ARE DANGEROUS. The only reason the man lost the suit was because, when the amalgam material is shipped to the dentists, it carries a WARNING.

More recently a group filed a lawsuit against the FDA for failure to classify amalgam fillings as unsafe. FINALLY, on 5-29-08, U.S. FDA settled the lawsuit by agreeing to provide a WARNING about dental amalgams.

Now I ask you, why would the FDA fight this in the first place? Everyone in the world knows that Mercury is highly toxic.

The question is "Would you prefer to have dental fillings with or without poison?"

MSG (Monosodium Glutamate)

MSG is a dreadful food additive that causes much pain and suffering. Thousands of people have written complaint letters to the FDA and the FDA completely ignores them. MSG is basically a taste enhancer and tenderizer. It is a multi-billion dollar business today and you will find MSG, or some ingredient which includes MSG, in most of your processed foods in the market. The reason they use it is because they can use inferior foods and make them taste better with MSG.

Now, you're 'gonna' chuckle at this one, but it 'ain't' funny. Where do you think the scientists get fat rats for studies of obesity, diet, and diabetes? They create them by injecting newborn rats with MSG. They even have a name for them; "MSG-Treated Rats." This fact alone should tell you why obesity is an epidemic in our country. This should also tell you why you should avoid all foods containing MSG.

I could go on and on but if you're really interested in learning more, you may want to read the following two books written by MEDICAL DOCTORS:

"Excitotoxins, The Taste That Kills" by R.L. Blaylock, MD

"In Bad Taste, The MSG Syndrome" by George Schwartz, MD

MSG is well known as a cause of migraine headaches. It is also especially hazardous to children. MSG may cause many problems for children but especially Attention Deficit Disorder (ADD) and also mood changes such as depression and even suicide.

Aspartame

Aspartame is one of the most common sugar substitutes. You will also find it in many diet drinks.

I don't drink any soft drinks, but if I did, I have always thought that I would avoid the DIET drinks because all the people I see drinking them are fat. I don't want to be fat, so I would avoid diet drinks. Ha ha ha. Perhaps you will see a little humor in the cartoon I saw recently. This fat man was ordering in a fast food restaurant. He ordered a double cheeseburger, super sized French fries and A DIET COKE. The reason I think that is so funny is because aspartame has been proven to make you FATTER. Aspartame is one of the most dangerous food additives. Seventy-five percent of all the FDA consumer complaints are about aspartame. There are 92 different adverse symptoms including DEATH. The symptoms include headaches, memory loss, seizures, vision loss, coma and cancer.

Can you believe that people are drinking diet drinks because they are concerned about their weight, when actually they are making it worse? What more can I say?

The pH Miracle and Diet

A good diet is absolutely critical to your good health. A good diet will include all the necessary nutrients, vitamins and minerals and it should all be organic. That's the best way I know of to avoid MSG, aspartame and all the other poisons they add to our processed food. The FDA has approved over 25,000 food additives which are TOXIC. Now, any one of them might be all right, but 25,000 is a bit too much. Our bodies have an immune system to handle some toxins, but they cannot handle that volume.

Our bodies are highly sophisticated and require a large variety of foods. Nutrients are like building blocks. Every cell in your body is replaced about every seven years. Without these building blocks, that cannot happen. Again, a good diet is required.

A friend of mine is now taking a college course on nutrition taught by a doctor. In his introductory letter to all students he makes the statement that "Our population is becoming quite acidic and suffers also from chronic semi-dehydration." In other words, he is touting the very principles of pH and hydration.

All life exists or ceases to exist at the CELLULAR LEVEL. Your cells require an alkaline pH to function correctly. When you die, the body's pH immediately begins to turn from alkaline to acidic and the decaying process begins. So, when you are alive and you have an acidic pH, you have already begun the dying process. When your pH becomes acidic, the oxygen level drops and calcium is depleted and your electrical system no longer functions correctly. All types of unwanted pathogens love an acidic environment and they begin to thrive.

The pH factor is an indication of your diet and whether it's been good or bad. If your diet is too low in nutrients, your pH will be low. If your diet contains too many toxins, your pH will be low. If you have a mineral deficiency, your pH will be low. Are you getting the idea that a low pH is not good? Well, you're right. pH was one of the first things I learned about early in my search for treating my ALS condition. At that time, I was still pretty bad off with my ALS. I was very near the bottom of the scale; very weak and lethargic with very limited range of motion in my entire body.

When I first ordered my Coral Calcium supplement, they sent Dr. Barefoot's book and a pH test kit along with it. The test kit is a roll of litmus paper in a plastic container. They also included a paper explaining how to interpret the readings plus special instructions. The instructions said to test your saliva on the litmus paper, but only after not eating any food or drink for two hours. On the plastic container, they show the various colors of the litmus paper and their corresponding numerical rating. The range is from 6.0 through 8.0. Dead center is 7.0. Yellow is 6.0, green is 7.0, and blue is 8.0. If you are below 7.0, your body is acidic and you are sick. 7.0 is neutral. Any reading above 7.0 means you are alkaline and you should be healthy. Everything I have read about pH, says that 7.35 is normal.

"Eric, why are you going into all this detail?"

Because I don't want you to just read about it, I want you to get a real feeling for it. THIS IS IMPORTANT.

Remember I was really sick and my first pH test was off the chart; well below the 6.0 with a very pale yellow. Here is what the instructions said about my reading:

"If your pH is below 6.0, then you are highly acidic, very mineral deficient, and may have contracted at least one degenerative disease."

Now, let me ask you, does that hit the nail on the head or what? I was shocked by the accuracy of the pH test. I first thought to look for a comparison, so I had Glenna test her saliva. Well, guess what, her's was 7.3. I should not have to explain to you, but that made me a real believer about pH.

OK, so now I'm a real believer in pH, and I thought that anything in the area of 7.0 was all right. BUT, my experience tells me otherwise. My experience has convinced me that if you had a reading of 6.0, and you raised it to 6.5, you would feel better; and if you had a reading of 7.0 and raised it to 7.5, you would feel even better yet. First of all, I've been in the range of 7.0 to 7.5 for a long time now.

Up Your pH—(pun intended!)

Here's what happened to me recently. One morning a few months ago, I woke up and was bubbling over to get out of bed and attack the world. I really felt good. Naturally, I rushed into the kitchen table to find my pH test kit. I put my saliva on the little strip of paper and it turned blue in a minute. For the first time, I realized that the higher on the scale the better you were, AND the better you felt.

Normally, I check my pH every morning. Over the years, I have come to realize that I feel better when my pH is higher. But more importantly, I realize that when I FEEL better, I am better. When I am better, I mean much stronger.

Now, I don't know about you, but my conclusion is this:

BALANCING YOUR pH IS THE BEST KEPT HEALTH SECRET IN THE WHOLE WORLD.

It is so simple. It is a do-it-yourself test that costs pennies a day and tells you more than any other medical test ever does. Further, you know exactly what to do about it if you're low. There will be more about that in this chapter. Please understand that most doctors don't know this. I had a doctor tell me that I was perfect on all the lab tests and that included a pH reading of 5.0. So, what did he know? Well, not much about pH.

Now, I always thought 7.0 or slightly higher was alkaline and just great. However, this new experience tells me that when you're 8.0, you're even better than anything less than that. The author of the book "The pH Miracle" says that around 7.5 is normal. However, I believe 8.0 is even better.

Most people don't know anything about pH and those who do know about it probably don't realize its true significance. My own personal experience with my pH has taught me a lot. I now believe almost everything I've read about pH in books written by MD's and/or nutritionists is true.

Your pH must be alkaline (well above a 7.0).

People with low or acidic pH are usually mineral deficient especially in calcium. Linus Pauling (the vitamin C guy) said that MINERAL DEFICIENCY is coincidental with ALL ILLNESS.

If you are looking for an anti-depressant, this is a really good one. The higher your alkaline level, the better you will feel. If your pH level is between 7.5 and 8.0, you will feel alive and enthusiastic about life. I would be willing to make you a small wager that most people on anti-depressant drugs probably have a low pH (acidic well below a 7.0). I believe it would be a good idea to check your pH BEFORE ever taking an anti-depressant drug. Of course, I don't believe in anti-depressant drugs anyway, except for EXTREME cases. Remember, drugs are toxic and all toxins will lower your pH.

You will find a list of alkaline and acidic foods at the end of the next chapter.

THIS COULD BE THE SINGLE MOST IMPORTANT FACTOR FOR YOUR GENERAL HEALTH—YOUR pH!

You might want to order a pH test kit right now before you forget. Call the number below; it only costs about $10.

(800) 899-8349

You will find a very interesting discussion about balancing your pH on the following web site:

http://www.evenbetternow.com/alkalize.asp

Raw Milk

Raw milk is what you get straight from the cow; un-homogenized and not even pasteurized. Now, common sense must tell you that raw milk must be better for you. That's why more and more people are switching to raw milk. There was a big article in the Health Section of the "Los Angeles Times" on March 2, 2009. In this article, they discuss the pros and cons of raw milk. Federal officials maintain that milk should be pasteurized to avoid the risk of contamination. What I think that really means is that producers of raw milk must maintain more SANITARY conditions. They also say there's no proven benefit to drinking raw milk. But, in my opinion, that's simply not true. Everyone should know that when you cook or heat any raw food, you will destroy some of the nutrients in the food. If you are lucky like I was, your mother fed you on breast milk which is raw milk. I think most people know that mother's milk is far better than any other milk. I talked to an ALS patient just the other day who had survived ALS for 15 years (almost as long as I have). He claimed that whey protein was responsible for a lot of his physical improvement. Now, get this. Not just any whey protein, but only whey protein made from raw milk. I should say raw, organic milk. My conclusion is that raw milk is one of the best foods available to man. Remember, babies survive and grow living on nothing but milk for the first several months of their lives. It must be good.

Sunshine

Get out in the sunshine several times a week for a minimum of thirty minutes to an hour. By the way, the sun does not cause cancer, but sunscreens do. They are toxic and prevent you from getting vitamin D. Sunshine is a natural anti-depressant. Research proves that countries where people are exposed to high levels of UVB from the sun have LOWER cancer rates. These are countries located in the tropics. Also, cancer rates increase as blood levels of vitamin D decrease. If you cannot get out in the sunshine enough, then you could consider taking vitamin D as a supplement. However, make sure it is vitamin D-3. You may consider taking up to 4,000 or 5,000 mg and maybe as much as 10,000 mg of vitamin D-3 daily, depending on how much you are exposed to sunshine.

"The Los Angeles Times" newspaper reported on 6-10-08 the following:

"A study released today found that men who are deficient in the so-called sunshine vitamin—vitamin D—have more than double the normal risk of suffering a heart attack." They also said that another new study "found that low levels of vitamin D increased the risk of diabetes." A third study "linked deficiency to an increased risk of dying from breast cancer." My conclusion is that sunshine or vitamin D is critical to good health and does more to prevent illness than any drug could ever do.

Diet

You already know I like logic. Assuming you want to live a long and healthy life, what should you LOGICALLY do? I suggest that you look at how our ancestors lived and what they ate or drank for openers. This should provide you with some fundamentals. There are many, but let's talk about just two of them; water and meat.

Our ancestors drank only water; not one or two or maybe ten or twelve Coke's, Pepsi's or other carbonated drinks. Nowadays, most people drink too many bottled sodas and not enough pure water. Water is good and we should drink more. Water bottled in glass is better than tap water for one simple reason. It usually does not contain chlorine or fluoride. They are both toxic and they're both carcinogens. The simple question is this: "Would you prefer your drinking water with or without poison?"

What about meat? Many nutritionists believe we should be vegetarians. Our ancestors were not vegetarians and we should not be either. We know that from the animal bones found in their caves where they lived, and we know that because of our canine-like teeth. Although they have receded from previous generations, we still have four teeth in our mouths which are pointed. These teeth are called canines. Only carnivorous creatures have canine teeth.

According to one book that I read, there were over twenty species of humanoids on this planet and only one of them survived; the Homo sapiens (that's us). Scientists believe that we out-survived all the other humanoids because our brains became more developed providing a higher level of intelligence. More importantly the scientists believe that this happened because our diet INCLUDED MEAT. Meat was therefore highly significant in our evolution. When we say meat that probably means a lot of fish. Scientists know from DNA studies that we evolved from one small tribe in Africa. As we grew in numbers and spread throughout the world, we always followed the shoreline. Apparently we loved the water and maybe we loved fish and other seafood. Incidentally, that's probably why we have little or no hair on our bodies. Mammals living in the ocean have no hair. Most land mammals, other than us, have very hairy bodies.

A recent survey by the National Institutes of Health of almost 500,000 people who ate more than 3 oz. to 5 oz. of meat daily had a far greater risk of cancer. However, the study included all types of meat such as sausage, bologna, bacon and other PROCESSED meat. An entirely different study indicated that red meat such as steak or prime rib did not cause cancer. I remember reading another article a long time ago about sausage. There was a small town in Europe where the men had a very high incidence of heart attacks and cancer. Coincidentally, the town's major industry was a sausage factory. Most of the men in town thought it was "macho" to eat a lot of sausage and they included it in every meal. What does that tell you? I've never seen a study on organic red meat (not processed meat). I'm fairly certain that a study like that would prove red meat is good for you. Meat has many nutrients not found in other foods.

My conclusion about meat in our diet is this; it should be included. However, we should eat more vegetables and less meat. We probably need fish in our diet at least once or twice a week. Warning: You better avoid all fish unless you are certain they contain no Mercury.

Prescription Eye Glasses

When you realize you may need glasses, that may be your first indication that you have a nutritional deficiency. That may be corrected by eating more nutritious food and adding a B-Complex supplement and Glyconutrients. Also eggs are very beneficial for your eyes.

Organic Food

Organic food is the fastest growing segment in the food industry and for good reason.

We now have two large supermarkets in our area providing us with a large number of organic food items and a tremendous variety. They even have organic ice cream; can you believe that?

You might be wondering why organic? Well, it is really quite simple. Most of the food in regular markets contains many toxins including MSG, Aspartame and preservatives. Not only that, but they are now modifying our food to make it more insect resistant and that means it's more toxic. Also, they are irradiating our food to reduce bacteria development after being harvested. That's great, but irradiation also destroys the vitamins and minerals in the food.

While we are talking about irradiation, warming or cooking your food in the microwave is not the best way to go. I have read that blood must be warm before it can be transfused, but if you use a microwave to warm it, it will kill the patient. Also, food in a plastic container should not be warmed or cooked in the microwave because the toxins in the plastic may transfer to the food.

Now that you know all this, let me ask you one simple question:

"Would you like your meals with or without poison and with or without nutrients?"

I don't think I need to offer any further comments. That fairly well sums it up, don't you think?

Plastic Containers with Food and Water

An e-mail was sent to me with a subject of "Cancer update." This story would tend to support the theory that most any toxin can cause cancer. The e-mail said Sheryl Crow was on the "Ellen Show" and said that she developed breast cancer from leaving bottled water in her car. The e-mail went on to explain that we should never leave our bottled drinking water in plastic contains in our car that may be subject to high temperatures. Plastic contains toxins and the heat causes the toxins to leak into the water.

Actually, I think you should not store food or water in plastic containers and then freeze them or heat them. This is only my opinion, but I think it may be all right to store food and water in plastic as long as you don't heat or freeze it while in the plastic container.

Styrofoam cups should never be used to serve hot coffee or any hot drink. Styrofoam is an oil-based product containing carcinogens.

Smoking Tobacco

Anyone with a working brain should know that smoking is detrimental to your health. It is probably the second DUMBEST thing we do. Before you get mad at me, I smoked cigarettes for about ten years so I was dumb too. Here is a short story about smoking:

My stepdad, George, smoked two or three packs a day all of his life and he started at age 13. He always had one in his mouth. At about age 65, he developed Emphysema and that is a horrible disease with no cure. One day as he was leaving the doctor's office, the doctor said *"George, why don't you stop on your way home and buy some rat poison?"* George said *"What for?"* The doc said *"Because that would be quicker."* The doc meant the rat poison would be quicker than continuing to smoke cigarettes.

Later when George wound up in a nursing home, I called him one day to chat. George told me that his breathing was so bad he had to sit down and rest halfway through a shower. I said *"That's the shits."* He said *"It's worse than that."* I will never forget his response.

Sometimes we just don't realize just how bad, "bad" can be. So, if you smoke now, I would urge you to quit. There are too many health problems that are caused by smoking. Tobacco contains toxins.

Obesity and Overweight

I've read that two-thirds of us are overweight and half of those are obese. This is probably our biggest health problem in the country today. Overweight people will develop many other health problems. There are many foods and food additives that contribute to this problem and could be avoided. They will be mentioned later on in this chapter. Other than that, I have an idea that might shed some light on why we have this problem. This is something that I've never read anywhere else but I believe in it based on my own 79 years of experience. Question: Why do some people CRAVE certain fattening foods? Here is what I think happens. When a person does not eat NUTRITIOUS food, the body's taste buds will change and the body will demand more food.

When I drank my first cup of coffee at age 16, I thought it was awful. I had to add cream and three spoons of sugar just to make it palatable. Later on in life, I learned to enjoy coffee without any additives. Then, along came decaf. When I drank my first cup, my taste buds said this is just like regular coffee. BUT, after two or three days, my taste buds said "Oh no it isn't." I think what happens is your body tells you real coffee is good only because it gives you a lift. Did you know that coffee is considered a drug because of that?

This is only one example. I think the same thing happens with sugar. When your body does not have a wholly satisfying diet of nutritious food, it welcomes anything that will give it a lift. Sugar will definitely give you a temporary increase in energy. This may develop into a craving for all foods containing sugar.

Most overweight people have cravings for certain foods. My theory is that this is the heart of the problem and if we could eliminate the cravings, we would not be overweight. The second part of my theory is that the cravings are caused by nutritional deficiency. In other words, if you feed your body properly, that is a diet of highly nutritional foods, and then you will not have cravings.

I am not overweight and I believe my body reacts normally. The reason I say that is because I like pie and ice cream just like anyone else, but I also love good fresh vegetables. Simply put, I believe that if you follow a diet of a lot of fresh vegetables and fruits, you are much less apt to develop a craving for any of the wrong kinds of foods like sugar.

Allowing ourselves to become fat is the third dumbest thing we do. We know the cause so it is easily prevented or corrected. If you think you are unable to lose weight, let me remind you of this fact. I've seen many pictures of the Holocaust victims and I have never seen a fat person. If you really want to be healthy, then you must maintain a normal weight.

At this point, you might be wondering why I told you smoking was the second dumb thing we do and being overweight is the third. You are probably wondering what is the first dumb thing we do? Well, in my opinion, the number one dumb thing we do as a society is we continue to allow our medical doctors to prescribe drugs which do not CURE our illness. Taking most prescription drugs and anticipating a cure is just a little short of insanity.

This is the end of things to KNOW and the next will be things to DO.

CHAPTER 15

PREVENTION
PART THREE—THINGS TO DO

This is all about things to DO which may prevent illness and for treatment of MINOR illnesses. If you have a really serious or life-threatening illness, then you may need to see a medical doctor. Nothing in here is meant to cure any illness. Remember, I am not a doctor and I have no medical training. These are things that have either worked for me or that I believe may help others based on what I have read by health care professionals. I am not recommending anything in here because we are all different. What works for me may not work for you. You should consult with your health care professional. No, I did not say medical doctor. They probably will not agree with my thoughts.

Preventing Illness with the Three-D Program

There are many things you can do to make yourself healthier and avoid illness. I think you can prevent most sickness with a Three-D Program of Detoxification, Diet, and the D vitamin or sunshine. These three items plus exercise may improve your health.

Here are some suggestions:

Detoxification and Avoiding Toxins

The very first and most important thing to do is consider the removal of all your Silver (Mercury) dental fillings (amalgams). It is my suggestion that you do this BEFORE doing any other form of detoxification.

You might also be wise to eliminate ALL metal dental fillings and all root canal teeth. You must find a dentist who is experienced in amalgam removal and will take all the necessary precautions during removal.

Some dentists may charge thousands of dollars for amalgam replacement. You don't have to pay that much. Check around. In 1998, my dentist charged me approximately $125 each to remove my two amalgam fillings and replace them with porcelain.

Call DAMS and request their free INFORMATION KIT. The kit will include a wealth of information about dental work, specific instructions on amalgam removal, and a list of dentists in your area.

DAMS, Inc.

Phone (651) 644-4572

E-mail: dams@usfamily.net

I highly recommend a Huggins-trained dentist:

http://www.drhuggins.com/default.asp?PageName=Alliance%20Members

A Huggins-trained dentist can provide you with a Compatibility Report based on your blood test. This Compatibility Report will tell you what metals and other types of crowns, fillings, etc. that are most compatible with your system.

Bowel Movements

Avoiding constipation may be the second most important thing of any detoxification program. I would suggest that you consider having a few colon hydrotherapy treatments before any other detox treatments. It is also a good idea to have one immediately following any detox treatment. Toxins cause cancer and many other illnesses. Frequent BM's will help the body eliminate rather than retain toxins. According to what I've read, two or three BM's daily may also help. I drink two spoonfuls of Psyllium in a 12 oz. glass of water before breakfast and dinner. Psyllium is a natural colon cleanse and an assist for bowel regularity. Occasional colon hydrotherapy treatments are a great idea.

Detoxifying Your Body

Heavy metals, pesticides, and toxic pathogens especially those in your colon can cause health problems. They should be removed to obtain maximum health. There are many ways to detox including Bentonite clay baths, Ionic foot baths, DMPS Chelation (primarily for Mercury), EDTA Chelation (primarily for Lead), infrared saunas, Chlorine Dioxide and take cilantro or chlorella.

There are some new methods for detox that I have not tried, but all that I've read indicates to me that they work. Phospholipid and Glutathione Infusion are both good. Also, vitamin C ascorbates and a product called OSR they say can boost your body's own production of Glutathione. Vitamin D may help detox.

Glutathione

Our bodies produce Glutathione naturally. It may be the best detoxifier known. You may have your doctor provide you with Glutathione by IV, or better yet, take some supplement like Liposomal liquid that causes the body to produce more Glutathione. Also, asparagus may produce Glutathione.

Bentonite Clay Baths

One of my favorite methods of detoxification is the Bentonite clay baths or foot baths.

You may order Bentonite clay from Even Better Now. All the instructions come with your order of the clay.

To order online go to:
http://www.evenbetternow.com/clay-baths.php
To order by phone, call toll free
(877) 562-6039
Questions and International Orders call
(520) 877-2637

Locating a Doctor for Chelation Treatments by IV (ACAM Doctor)

The American College for Advancement in Medicine (ACAM) is a not-for-profit medical society. Most of these doctors do Chelation treatments. However, not all of them have the same degree of Chelation training. You still must be selective in your choice of a doctor.

ACAM represents more than 1,000 physicians in many countries. To find one in your area, you can look at the web site below or call:

The American College for Advancement in Medicine
23121 Verdugo Dr., Suite 204

Laguna Hills, CA 92653
Phone (949) 583-7666 or Toll Free Outside CA (800) 532-3688
http://www.acam.org/

Hair Analysis

Here is one health test that I recommend which is relatively inexpensive. A hair analysis will tell you if you are low in necessary minerals and also if you're high in unwanted toxic heavy metals such as Mercury, Arsenic, etc.

See your doctor or health care professional for a hair analysis. They can order one from:

Great Smokies Diagnostic Lab
63 Zillicoa Ave.
Asheville, NC 28801
Phone (828) 253-0621

Most medical doctors don't know about hair analyses, so here's a better way to get your hair analysis:

Call Dr. Kathleen Akin
Phone (800) 528-4223 or see the web site below:
http://www.advancedfamilyhealth.com/index.htm

Klinghardt and Detox Information

Here is a really great web site for more information on detox treatments:

For more information about detox, do a search for KLINGHARDT. That will bring up many web sites. Click on the fifth one down *"Nine Steps, etc."*

http://www.hbci.com/~wenonah/new/9steps.htm

Diet

THE MAIN THING ABOUT A HEALTHY DIET IS THAT IT INCLUDES MORE ALKALINE FOOD AND LESS ACIDIC FOOD, AND ALSO THAT IT BE ALL ORGANIC.

A nutritious diet is made of a variety of fresh ORGANIC fruits, vegetables, and nuts. A large portion should be raw. There should be limited meat and no fish (unless Mercury free). A good diet should be free of all toxins especially MSG and aspartame.

Eliminate Toxins in Your Environment

Eliminate all sources of toxins in your environment, especially in your home. There are so many toxins in your environment that I am unable to list them all. I can only give you a general idea of what they are. I have read that the air in your home may be five times more polluted than the air outside. This pollution is caused by toxic household cleaners, insect sprays, deodorizers, laundry detergent, wood paneling, wood flooring, hair sprays, upholstered furniture, carpeting, and even computers and TVs which have been sprayed with fire retardant. Also, many cosmetics, aftershave, perfume, nail polish and nail polish removers, and other body lotions may contain toxins. Tap water in your home usually contains chlorine and sometimes fluoride. These are both carcinogens and are known to cause cancer and more. The number of toxic things in our homes is unbelievable; even most toothpastes are toxic.

Chlorine Dioxide

Chlorine dioxide may help you improve your pH. Some people say that chlorine dioxide is the most effective killer of pathogens known to man and can even kill a virus. The medical establishment does not know about this and has no drug that will do the same thing. Chlorine dioxide is approved by the Environmental Protection Agency for safely removing pathogens and contaminates like anthrax. It is slowly replacing chlorine for municipal water treatment systems. The American Society of Analytical Chemists proclaimed in 1999 that chlorine dioxide is the most powerful pathogen killer known to man. Normal levels of oxygen in the blood cannot destroy all the pathogens, but chlorine dioxide is one part chlorine and two parts oxygen.

Chlorine dioxide is said to kill almost any virus such as hepatitis, HIV, bird flu, malaria, colds, and the flu. Based on my experience using chlorine dioxide, I believe that is true. You might want to consider ordering chlorine dioxide and just keep it around.

NO ANTIBIOTIC DRUG THAT I KNOW OF WILL KILL A VIRUS. Remember, colds and the flu are both caused by a virus.

For more information, go to your computer and do a "Search" for chlorine dioxide.

Colloidal Silver

Colloidal Silver is a natural antibiotic and has been known to effectively eliminate unwanted pathogens from your colon. Colloidal Silver is a selective killer of pathogens and relatively harmless to other cells in the body. Most of us have excessive bad bacteria, fungus, and/or mycoplasmas in our colons.

If you are interested in making your own Colloidal Silver, there is a unit you can buy for about $200 US:

The SilverGen SG6 Automatic Colloid Generator

Phone (877) 745-8374 or (360) 732-5091

http://www.silvergen.com/

You may want to order a COLLOIDAL SILVER MANUAL. It costs about $70 but it's probably worth a great deal more for all of its benefits. It's the only source of information on dosage that I know of.

Call this number to order it: (866) 888-8628

For more information, go to your computer and do a "Search" for Colloidal Silver.

By the time you read this, the above items may no longer be available. Never underestimate the power of money.

Hydrogen Peroxide

You can buy "35% Food Grade Hydrogen Peroxide" at your health food store—do not use regular peroxide, it may contain heavy metals—do not use full strength. Best to drink on an empty stomach so the oxygen goes into the bloodstream and kills virus/bacteria/fungus, etc. This is another effective detoxifier.

Add 32 drops peroxide to one quart distilled water. You can slowly build up to 100 drops per quart of water by increasing one drop per day. You may consider drinking one to three quarts a day.

For more information, go to your computer and do a "Search" for peroxide.

Headline News

If Big Pharma were to develop a drug that would kill a virus, it would make headlines. BUT, they already have natural elements that will kill a virus. That should be headline news, but very few people know that. Remember, the flu is caused by a virus and if we had a cure for the flu it would make flu vaccinations a thing of the past. I'm almost certain that chlorine dioxide and Colloidal Silver will kill a virus. I think peroxide will also do that. The reason I'm telling you all this is because you may benefit from this information. If you are wise, you would do what Glenna and I have already done. We purchased a ten-year supply of chlorine dioxide and we own a SilverGen SG6 Automatic Colloid Generator. When we feel a cold developing, we immediately take chlorine dioxide or Colloidal Silver and WE DO NOT get a cold. We also keep a small amount of Colloidal Silver in a spray bottle. We always spray it on any cut to prevent infection. You spray it on and let it air dry. This should avoid infections like MRSA.

Prescription Drugs

Avoid taking prescription drugs long-term. Drugs can be of great benefit for emergencies and other short-term applications. Taking one or more toxic drugs long-term and expecting your health to improve is just short of insanity. Vitamin D, for one example, can do more to prevent heart attacks than all the heart drugs could ever do including those that lower cholesterol.

Here is one example: If a man needs Viagra for E. D., there is an underlying physical problem and the cause of E. D. Studies have proven that E. D. is a forerunner of heart attacks. Instead of Viagra, I would try Testosterone. Testosterone requires a prescription, but it is a natural hormone, not a drug. Also, you might try Ribose or L-arginine. Here is a special note for guys that need Viagra: If you are also concerned about "size matters," then whatever you do, don't use Crisco on it because that's shortening. Ha Ha

Many situations call for the use of an antibiotic. However, before I would take a drug antibiotic, I would try natural antibiotics such as chlorine dioxide, peroxide, Colloidal Silver, garlic, olive leaf extract or oil of oregano.

In addition to all of the above, here are some health tips:

This is just another reminder that I'm not a doctor and I'm not even a nutritionist. These health tips are simply what I believe in.

Sugar

Minimize your use of sugar. Use Stevia Leaf Extract instead. Another one is Xylitol. Stevia is my personal preference of all the sugar substitutes—non-toxic.

Avoid HFCS (high-fructose corn syrup)

This is a sweetener used in many food and drink products. Studies have shown that it depresses thyroid function and lowers one's metabolic rate. HFCS will increase fat and destroy your health.

Pies and Pastries

Avoid or minimize flour and foods that are primarily flour and/or sugar.

Cooking Oils

Avoid most cooking oils. For one example, I have read that canola oil is an industrial oil and not fit for human consumption. Use olive oil and coconut oil.

Butter Substitutes

Avoid margarine and all other butter substitutes—some BUTTER IS GOOD for you.

Carbonated Drinks

Avoid carbonated drinks. Many of them contain toxic ingredients and carbon dioxide is also toxic. Plain water is good. Avoid DIET drinks especially as many of them contain aspartame.

Tobacco

Avoid cigarettes and all tobacco.

Watch Your Weight

Avoid being overweight. You simply can't be fat and expect to live a long and healthy life. Sugar and starch make fat. One hundred years ago, we were lean and the average annual sugar consumption per person was five pounds. Today it's over 150 pounds. Sugar causes diabetes as well as weight gain. Avoid starch foods like white bread, white rice, white potatoes and white pasta. Avoid aspartame and MSG. Starvation diets do not work because the body's metabolism slows down and saves fat. If you do not follow a NUTRITIOUS diet, your body does the same thing. A moderate nutritious alkaline diet of three or four smaller meals a day is suggested. Avoid eating when you are not hungry. If you're not hungry at your normal mealtime, it means you ate too much at your last meal.

Although all calories are not created equally, there is something to be said about shear volume of food. I think it is a good idea to fill your plate one time based on what you know to be a reasonable amount of food for you. THEN, DO NOT HAVE SECONDS. One more thing that my mother taught me years ago: Do not eat in between meals.

Obesity can take two to ten years off your life expectancy.

Weight Control

Avoid the "See Food" Diet—that's when you SEE FOOD and you EAT FOOD.

The BATHROOM SCALE is possibly the most effective weight control device ever invented. Weigh yourself EVERY morning upon first arising. Do this one year and you will be amazed at what happens.

You might try eating one half of a grapefruit before each meal.

Health Tonic & Weight Control

Here is another tip that may help you. A little bit of vinegar, lime juice and cinnamon before you eat can be very effective for weight loss. Before each meal eat one tablespoon of apple cider vinegar, 1/4 or less teaspoon of cinnamon and about one teaspoon of lime juice. Buy REAL cinnamon at the health food store. It must be UNFILTERED APPLE CIDER vinegar and that will also help your pH be more alkaline. This may cause loose stool or mild diarrhea at first. It should not last more than three days. Hang in there and you'll be glad you did.

Water

The water we drink should be as pure as possible. Distilled water is about as pure as it gets, but it contains no minerals. Most water filters remove most minerals also. We must have a source of quality minerals to be healthy. Possibly the best drinking water is natural spring water from a source that is pure and which contains minerals naturally. You may want to do a "Search" on the Internet for "mineral water" and see what you find. I've also learned that bathing or showering in chlorinated water is not a good idea either. You may absorb more chlorine bathing than if you drank it. You may want a water purifier.

Alcohol

Limit alcohol consumption to one or two drinks daily.

Coffee

Limit coffee consumption to one or two cups daily

Exercise

Even as little as ten minutes a day will do wonders for your health. Exercise has many health benefits. You need two types of exercise: Brisk walking or jogging alternately, to boost your heart rate and weight bearing exercises primarily for the upper body to maintain strength. Muscles atrophy from lack of use. An old axiom is *"USE IT OR LOSE IT."* Exercise in conjunction with a nutritious diet will have synergistic benefits.

It is very difficult to develop an exercise habit. Here is what I did. I learned about the 30-day rule. If you want to develop a new habit, you should establish a schedule of time of day for your new exercise. Then you do it everyday according to your schedule for 30 days and it will become a habit. If you miss one day, then you start over. You must do it for 30 CONSECUTIVE days. One thing very important, in the beginning make your exercise very short and simple so there's no excuse for not doing it. I decided I wanted to run or jog every morning before work, but only on work days and not on the weekend. I made my exercise very short and simple; I just ran around the block which took about three minutes. Then after 30 days, I began to make my run longer. It was all very easy.

I HAVE TRIED ALL OF THE FOLLOWING FOODS AND SUPPLEMENTS AND I BELIEVE THEY HAVE SPECIAL VALUE. REMEMBER, I AM A LIVING TEST LAB, BUT ALSO REMEMBER WE ARE ALL DIFFERENT. What has worked for me may not work for you.

Take Healthy Supplements of Vitamins and Minerals

Buy only the very best vitamin/mineral supplements which are natural (no synthetic) and pure (non-toxic). Parting with your money for health supplements is an investment, not an expense. There's no better way to spend your money than on your health. For basics, I would suggest the following: A good multi-vitamin/mineral, B complex, vitamin E, and antioxidants like A and C, plus Co-Q-10. Also, the sunshine vitamin D. Another good one is Niacinamide. One of the more important supplements is GLYCONUTRIENTS. Additionally, our bodies need adequate minerals in our water, food or in a supplement. It just may be that minerals are equally important to vitamins; maybe even more important.

I believe it is important to take vitamins that are PURE and non-toxic. You will find that today they have vitamins that are beyond organic, that are made from natural raw (uncooked) food, gluten free, dairy free and 100% active ingredients (no fillers or binders).

Fruits and Vegetables

Eat much of your fruits and vegetables RAW—you may want to use a juicer. Eat a lot of greens.

Eat apples and bananas often—maybe even everyday. They each provide many nutrients. Bananas are high in Potassium. (There is more about Potassium and Salt later in this chapter.)

"If an apple a day keeps the doctor away, then a banana a day will keep the surgeon at bay."

Eggs

They are an excellent food. There is no clear evidence that cholesterol is harmful. 80% of your cholesterol is produced by your body. It just can't be all bad. Lowering cholesterol will increase your risk of cancer and will not prevent heart attacks; that's my opinion. Eggs are really good for your eyesight. They can even help prevent macular degeneration which is a major cause of blindness.

Pomegranate Juice

A few ounces everyday provides benefits for your brain and nervous system. It may also lower blood pressure.

Cranberry Juice

Cranberries are good for fevers, gastrointestinal problems, and any swelling or inflammation. They are also known to fight urinary tract infections and gut infections as well as gum disease. They are also good for heart disease and cancer.

Lima Beans

The lima bean is a cousin to the soy bean. The soy bean is well noted for its health benefits. My own experience has taught me that lima beans are really good to raise your pH level. We buy frozen organic green lima beans and keep them on hand because we eat them often.

Turmeric

If this was a drug, it would be considered a "wonder drug" for all the health benefits.

Cayenne Pepper

This is another excellent food supplement with many health benefits.

Niacinamide

Many of our physical and mental health problems may be attributed to a deficiency of Niacinamide. I cannot tell you enough about the importance of this vitamin. You may want to read Dr. David Williams February 2009 "_Alternatives,_" a monthly health newsletter. Call this number: (800) 718-8293.

If you or someone you know has Alzheimer's, you really must read this article.

Cilantro

This is a natural detoxifier, especially for Mercury.

Chlorella

Chlorella is green algae containing chlorophyll, vitamins, minerals, dietary fiber, nucleic acids, amino acids, enzymes and more. Chlorella contains a growth factor and can stimulate healing. It will also improve your pH and it is a detoxifier. Spirulina is a similar product.

Asparagus

The information I have reviewed about asparagus has almost convinced me that it may prevent cancer. It may be another "wonder drug." It may include Glutathione or it may cause your body to produce more. It also may be a really great treatment and maybe even be a possible cure for kidney disease. You may want to use the following for prevention or treatment:

The asparagus must be cooked and then placed in a blender and liquefied to make a puree. Take four full tablespoons of the puree twice daily. You may take it hot or cold and diluted or not.

Lemon Juice

The lemon has long been considered medicine. Both of us take one teaspoon of pure fresh lemon juice twice a day in our water and that helps maintain an alkaline pH. Incidentally, while the lemon may be acidic, it DOES NOT make your body acidic.

Honey

Honey is an excellent food providing many benefits such as antioxidants and much more. Manuka honey is my preference and I eat about one heaping tablespoon everyday. I haven't had a cold or the flu for years. Be healthy—eat your honey.

Hydrogen Peroxide

A daily mouth rinsing with half water and half food grade hydrogen peroxide may prevent gum disease and gum infections.

Probiotics

Take probiotics and eat fermented food such as sauerkraut. Prescription drug antibiotics destroy GOOD BACTERIA in your colon. Probiotics and fermented food replace the good bacteria.

Immune System Boost

There are many products that supposedly will boost your immune system.

The ones I like and that may be good to prevent or treat colds are: Turmeric, vitamin C, cinnamon, ginger, Zinc, garlic and onions.

Fiber

One hundred years ago, most people had at least two BM's (bowel movements) everyday and they had a lot more fiber in their diet than we do today. I use a product which is 100% Psyllium husk for my fiber and I have two BM's everyday without fail. I take one heaping teaspoon and one level teaspoon in a glass of pure water twice a day; one before breakfast and one before dinner. It is best to drink your water at least ten minutes before a meal.

Starbucks Chai Tea Latte

I drank coffee for years and years and then I discovered that too much of it caused my anxiety attacks. I searched for a good substitute for a long time and then finally found this Starbucks drink. Now I am hooked more than I ever was on coffee. I have been drinking this almost everyday for about four years. Frequently I feel much stronger about two or three hours after my latte. I drink a 20 oz. Venti chai tea latte with soy milk. Much has been written about whether soy is good or bad. My opinion is that it's good and that's not my theory, but my experience. I know it's good for me. Maybe it's really the ginger, black tea, honey and cinnamon that's in the chai tea. Incidentally, I understand that they only use ORGANIC soy milk. I think that's great. At any rate, I don't want to live one day without my soy chai latte. I just learned that tea contains L-theanine and L-theanine boosts energy and concentration.

Preventing Heart Attacks

Nattokinase NSK-SD

This is a supplement that I believe can dissolve blood clots. This could possibly prevent heart attacks and strokes caused by blood clots. It is a derivative of the soy bean.

Nitric Oxide

Follow a diet to cause your body to produce more Nitric Oxide and at the same time the diet should improve your pH to more alkaline. Also, you may want to add a supplement MTHF which is a biologically active form of folic acid and will also increase your body's Nitric Oxide.

Chelation with EDTA

This is one of the best treatments for improving the condition of your entire circulatory system. I have talked to many people who have had this treatment and they all swear by it.

Sardines

Eat only genuine sardines, not any small canned fish they may call sardines. They could add years to your life. Most people have a shortage of Omega 3 fatty acids. Sardines are an excellent source.

Omega-3 Fatty Acid

Many times I have read that we are all short of necessary Omega-3 fatty acids. If you are unable to eat sardines, then you may want to add fish oil or soy oil to your diet because they are both good sources of Omega-3. They also help your body produce more Glutathione and all this is good for your heart.

Chia Seeds

This is a highly nutritious food. Chia is the richest known vegetable source of Omega-3 fatty acids. Another ALS person wrote to me about the tremendous improvement he had from eating chia seeds. The seeds also contain six concentrated antioxidants.

Cinnamon

1/4 teaspoon (or less) cinnamon daily can benefit your heart and circulation. Some cinnamon in the regular markets may be a fake cinnamon. You might want to buy real cinnamon at a health food store.

Lecithin

Lecithin is 10 times better for you than taking drugs to lower your cholesterol. From what I read, lecithin makes your blood more fluid and prevents a build up of plaque. Lecithin is a natural element found in RAW MILK and RAW EGGS. For that reason, I prefer my eggs with the yoke very runny because too much cooking will destroy the lecithin. Also, pasteurizing milk destroys the lecithin.

Eggplant Water

Here is an idea which may lower your blood pressure. Buy fresh organic eggplant and add six thin slices to two or three quarts pure drinking water and let soak overnight. Drink a quart or more everyday. It is pleasant tasting and can be substituted for any drinking water throughout the day.

Vitamin B-1 and Vitamin E

Both of these vitamins are beneficial to your circulatory system.

Resveratrol

The French outlive us by a few years and that may be primarily from drinking red wine. We now know the secret ingredient in wine is Resveratrol. This may help prevent heart attacks. The more I read about it, the more convinced I become that this is a very beneficial supplement. It not only increases your body's Nitric Oxide, but it can also inhibit the growth of cancer cells and even kill existing cancer cells.

Pomegranate Juice

Pomegranates or pomegranate juice is an excellent all-around food but especially beneficial for the heart and nervous system. Also, pomegranates, grapes, beets or beet juice, and Magnesium are known to reduce blood pressure.

Salt

Avoid excess salt. For several decades, salt has been linked to high blood pressure. Sprinkling a little salt on your eggs may not be the problem. The real problem is the heavy salt content in foods which are soaked in heavy salt brine such as bacon, pickles, olives and some processed meat such as bologna and hot dogs which contain excess salt. Also, cheese has a lot of salt.

Sodium (Salt) & Potassium Ratio

Here is a quote from the "Los Angeles Times" 2-23-09 *"A new study suggests that consuming twice as much potassium as sodium can halve your risk of dying from cardiovascular disease."* The article goes on to explain that the important factor is the ratio. In other words, it may not matter how much salt or how much potassium you have as long as the ratio of 2 to 1 is maintained. Now folks, that's BIG. Here is a natural treatment that can reduce heart problems by 50%. Remember, all the drugs to lower cholesterol have not reduced our heart attack rate. I'm sure the doctors will know about this and reduce their reliance on cholesterol drugs. Ha-ha-ha. Boy, is that funny or what? Don't hold your breath. I predict that will not happen anytime soon. The reason I say that is because I have known about this for over 40 years and so have some MD's. After my stepdad, George, had his third heart attack, he learned from his doctor about maintaining this balance between potassium and sodium. This balance kept George alive for another 25 years without another heart attack. You might remember I told you earlier that George died from emphysema.

*   *   *

It is our primary purpose to help people with their health problems and not to make money. You should understand that we have no financial interest in anything we have recommended or suggested. There is simply no profit motive on our part. All these ideas about foods and supplements are just what may help you and others with their health problems.

NOW, WE WANT TO REMIND YOU OF FOUR ITEMS OF REAL IMPORTANCE:

1. **If you are interested in our other book and/or more health information, you might visit this web site:**
    http://www.evenbetternow.com/als.asp

2. **Hair Analysis**
    Great Smokies Diagnostic Lab
    63 Zillicoa Ave.
    Asheville, NC 28801
    Phone (828) 253-0621
    Most medical doctors don't know about hair analyses, so here's a better way to get your hair analysis:
    Call Dr. Kathleen Akin
    Phone (800) 528-4223 or see the web site below:
    http://www.advancedfamilyhealth.com/index.htm

3. **pH Test Kit**
    You might want to order a pH test kit right now before you forget. Call the number below; it only costs about $10.
    Phone (800) 899-8349

4. **Dr. David Williams**
    You may want to call the number below for back issues of "Alternatives" by Dr. David Williams. They will send you a list of back issues.
    Phone (800) 718-8293

*   *   *

This chapter has provided you with much information that could help you be much healthier. We truly believe that you could add 10 or even 20 years to you life by just doing a few of these things. The main things are:

1. **Vitamin D (sunshine)**
2. **Maintain ratio of 2 to 1 potassium over sodium.**
3. **Avoid weight gain.**
4. **Avoid prescription drugs when possible.**
5. **Develop and maintain an alkaline pH.** This should be easy for most of you. Simply eliminate a few acidic foods and add a few alkaline foods to your daily diet. Eliminating and avoiding toxins may be necessary for some of you. A list of alkaline and acidic foods is provided below.

Alkaline & Acidic Foods

Alkaline Foods (The higher the number, the more alkaline)

Group 1 – (+1 thru +6)
Brussels sprouts +1, Asparagus +1, Lentils +1, Brazil nuts +1, Flax seeds +1, Olive oil +1, Buttermilk +1, Lettuce +2, Potato +2, Onion +3, Cauliflower +3, Tofu +3, Cabbage +4, Almonds +4, Flax seed oil +4, Peas +5, Sunflower seeds +5, Zucchini +6, Pumpkin +6
Group 2 – (+7 thru +14)
Spinach +8, Lime +8, Lemon +10, Carrot +10, Green string beans +11, Red beets +11, Lima beans +12, Soy beans +12, White navy beans +12, Garlic +13, Celery +13, Cabbage lettuce +14, Tomato +14, Bananas +14
Group 3 – (+15 or more)
Avocado +16, Red radish +16, Soy nuts +26, Barley grass +29, Soy sprouts +30, Alfalfa grass +30, Cucumber fresh +32, Wheat grass +34, Soy lecithin +38, Black radish +39

Acidic Foods (The higher the number, the more acidic)

Group 1 – (-1 thru –6)
Watermelon –1, Homogenized milk –1, Grapefruit –2, Cantaloupe –3, Liver –3, Rye bread –3, Cream –4, Butter –4, Strawberry –5, Plum –5, Whole-grain bread –5
Group 2 – (-7 thru –14)
Sunflower oil –7, Grape –8, Walnuts –8, Margarine –8, Honey –8, Papaya –9, Orange –9, Pear –10, Peach –10, Apricot –10, Wheat –10, White bread –10, Cashews –10, Fish, fresh water –12, Ketchup –12, Pineapple –13, Brown rice-13, Mayonnaise –13, Peanuts –13

<u>Group 3 – (-15 or more)</u>

Wine –16, Cheese –18, White sugar –18, Mustard –19, Fish, ocean –20, Chicken –20, Eggs –20, Chocolate –25, Coffee –25, Beer –27, Tea 27, Liquor –30, Fruit juice with sugar –33, Beef –34, Soy sauce –36, Pork –38, Vinegar –39

These items are the most common foods and were obtained from a more comprehensive list.

You might question some of the above ratings because I do. There may be a difference whether or not the food is organic. For example: Brown rice has a very low acidic rating, but I tested my organic brown rice and it is highly alkaline. You may want to know how to test your food. Of course you need a pH test kit. Some foods are acidic but make your body's pH more alkaline. For example: If you put a drop of pure fresh lemon juice directly on your test paper, it will test very acidic. BUT, if you put fresh lemon juice in your mouth and a few minutes later test your saliva, it will be highly alkaline. I've done this with my brown rice and it tests highly alkaline.

CHAPTER 16

PMA (POSITIVE MENTAL ATTITUDE)

No book about health would be complete without a discussion on PMA. All my successes in life, including my success at beating ALS, could only have come about through my PMA. If I did not have a positive attitude, I would not be alive today. When the doctor told me in 1995 that I would be dead in six months, I bought that idea but only for about one week. Then, I rekindled my PMA and began searching for what to do and eventually learned what to do. So, when you develop a health problem, I believe that you first must have or rekindle your PMA. You can't even drive a nail with a hammer unless you think you can do it. Am I right?

Life without pleasure and happiness is a wasted life in my opinion. Three things are required for happiness:

1. Something to do.
2. Something to look forward to.
3. Someone to love.

I believe you must have a positive attitude toward "something to do" and "something to look forward to." Also, you may never find someone to love if you do not have the right attitude.

There are two more things that are critical for happiness: You may want to get your bare skin out in the sun more often and follow an alkaline pH diet.

PMA is a powerful force and how it can work to your advantage is unknown to many people.

I can guarantee you that none of us, not even Einstein, know everything about life and our universe. PMA is one of those mysteries. Here is one proven indication that PMA has value. We know that people who live with pets, a dog or a cat, live longer lives than others. Now we know that's a fact, but again we don't thoroughly understand why. But it must have something to do with happiness and having a positive mental attitude and happiness are interrelated.

It is my belief that PMA, prayer, faith and hope are all the same thing or at least inseparably intertwined. The way you use your PMA is just the same way you would offer a prayer. You move to a secluded and quiet place to meditate. You think positively or pray to God about what you desire. You should first be thankful for what you have and do not ask for anything unreasonable. PMA or prayer may not always work as you probably know. It may have something to do with your karma or perhaps your method of thought. Whether it's prayer or PMA, I believe you must think about what you desire or pray for your desire OFTEN and with deep sincerity.

Let me give you just one example of how it works for me. Years ago, I made up a list of things that my wife and I wanted for our home such as a piano, wall-to-wall carpeting, etc. The list had about 10 items. I put the list in my shirt pocket which I wore to work everyday. I carried that list for about a year and there was no change. In other words, after about one year I had obtained nothing from that list even though I reviewed it often. So, what would any sensible person do at that point? Yes, you're right, I threw it away. About another year passed and I realized one day that I had obtained every item on that list. PMA or prayer does not always work overnight. Obviously, you must have a little patience.

If you are an Atheist or an Agnostic, I thoroughly understand because I was one of each of those at different times in my life. Perhaps the main thing I want to remind you of is that we simply DON'T KNOW everything about our universe. No one can say that they absolutely know everything about life on planet earth.

By now, you should have figured out that I like stories, and I have another one for you. The story will not prove anything except the fact that we don't know everything about our universe.

This story is about a curse put on the United States Presidents. Our ninth President, William Harrison, was sworn into office in January 1841. Somewhere along the way, William Harrison or the previous President did something to make one of our American Indian chiefs a bit upset to put it mildly. The Indian chief placed a curse on the White House. He said that President Harrison would die in office and every 20 years another President would die in office.

Now, you are probably like me, and I am highly skeptical of any curse and certainly one like this. However, that's just what happened. This is a story that just blows my mind and yet the facts are verifiable in the history books and on the Internet. Just do a search on the Internet for "U.S. Presidents." Let's go over the list of the Presidents who died in office.

William Harrison—Took office January 1841—Died April 4, 1841 of pneumonia.

Abraham Lincoln—Took office January 1861—Died April 15, 1865 after being shot.

James A. Garfield—Took office January 1881—Died September 19, 1881 after being shot.

William McKinley—Was re-elected to office in January 1901—Died September 4, 1901 after being shot.

Warren G. Harding—Took office January 1921—Died August 2, 1923 cause unknown.

Franklin D. Roosevelt—Was re-elected to office in January 1941—Died April 12, 1945 cause unknown.

John Kennedy—Took office January 1961—Died November 22, 1963 after being shot.

That's the end of the curse, but it is interesting that President Ronald Reagan took office in January 1981 and while in office he was shot and ALMOST died. Apparently that broke the curse.

Now I don't know what you think of all that, but I view that as the most astonishing story and thought provoking story that I have ever heard. Let's review the facts. Prior to the curse, no President had ever died while in office. Since the curse, seven Presidents have died while in office. Note that no other Presidents have died while in office except for these seven. Just in case you don't see how utterly remarkable this is, let me clarify one point. Whoever was President in January of 1841 and whoever was President 20 years later in January, died while in office. It seems to me that these seven occurrences are simply too great to be coincidental.

All of this does not prove anything, so you might be wondering why we included this story. We think it relates to PMA, God, prayer, faith, and hope. THIS STORY SHOULD PROVE TO YOU THAT WE CERTAINLY DO NOT KNOW EVERYTHING ABOUT LIFE. We think this relates especially to PMA and prayer. We cannot explain how the story about the presidents came about and we cannot explain how PMA and prayer works either, but we believe they do.

CHAPTER 17

SOLUTIONS FOR OUR MEDICAL SYSTEM

Problem

They say that if you do something the same way repeatedly and expect a different result, that is a form of insanity. Now that may apply to an individual, but it may also apply collectively to all of us. Here's what I mean. We as a nation are treating our illnesses almost exclusively with drugs and surgery. Many of us are unaware that most drugs do not cure, but we continue to take all these drugs expecting a cure. THAT IS INSANE.

There are many problems with our health care, but here is one that is overwhelming and fundamental. We have a large and growing number of sick people. If you double the number of sick people, as has happened in the past few decades, you also double the total COST of health care. Why is the U.S. one of the sickest countries in the world? Because our medical doctors are unable to provide cures. The reason for that is simple. Our doctors have been oversold on the value of prescription drugs to the extent that they seem to be avoiding most other types of treatments, and prescription drugs do not treat the cause and therefore do not provide a cure (with rare exceptions such as antibiotics).

The result is this; it is far too expensive and in spite of that, we are the sickest country in the world. Additionally, there are over 80 diseases for which the medical community has no cure. The real heart of the problem is that over half of the adult population in the U.S.A. has one or more chronic illnesses, and this number is growing.

WAKE UP AMERICA—The drug companies are not only killing us by the hundreds of thousands every year, but they are responsible for many problems with our medical care system. The drug companies virtually have nearly total control and they have FAILED US. Their drugs DO NOT CURE (with minor exceptions).

The heart of the problem is that our PROFIT-DRIVEN medical care system is focused only on PROFIT. There is literally no focus on CURING. No one is in charge of finding or investigating any cures. Our medical doctors appear to ignore all possible cures, at least that's my experience with my ALS and that appears to be uniform throughout our country. I have not heard of a new cure for any illness in the last 50 years.

News flash on TV channel CNBC on March 12, 2009—A new report by U.S. Business Roundtable stated that our medical care costs were so high that it was a LIABILITY TO THE GLOBAL ECONOMY. Doesn't that make you sit up and take notice? Is anyone in Congress reading this? It just may be time to correct this situation.

A major part of our problem is that we do not enjoy FREEDOM OF SPEECH when it comes to health care. If you make any statement that the drug companies do not like, the "Medical Mafia" may come after you and put you in jail or put you out of business. Frankly, I feel like I am taking my life in my own hands by publishing this book and that is not just an idle statement.

The USERS of MSG, Mercury dental fillings, and other toxic threats to our health tell us that these things make them sick. The SELLERS of these products say that they are perfectly safe. Who do you believe? Right now the court always believes the sellers because they have more money. That reminds me of THE GOLDEN RULE (not the one you're thinking of).

"THE ONE WITH THE MOST GOLD RULES."

Cause

The PRIMARY CAUSE of our medical care problem is that our medical doctors are not providing any cures. As a result we have too many sick people with chronic or incurable illnesses. Our medical doctors treat their patients almost exclusively with drugs and that is a result of BIG PHARMA HAVING TOO MUCH INFLUENCE ON OUR DOCTORS BEGINNING WITH MEDICAL SCHOOL. Most illnesses are caused by improper diet and exposure to toxins and our MD's are not trained to cope with that.

ALMOST ALL MEDICAL DOCTORS HAVE A STRONG PREFERENCE FOR PRESCRIPTION DRUGS AND THEY REFUSE

TO EVEN LOOK AT OR CONSIDER ANY ALTERNATIVE
TREATMENT. That would be OK except for the fact that MOST DRUGS
DO NOT CURE. Therefore, the only place you can look for any possible
cure is alternative treatment other than drugs.

If we have more and more patients, then the medical care costs go up
and up.

Many food additives such as MSG and Aspartame cause a multitude of
health problems. Most medical doctors don't seem to know about this.

Obesity is a major cause of health problems. I believe it is best treated
by diet but our MD's are not adequately trained to do that. They seem to
prefer prescribing drugs for all illness.

Nutritional deficiencies cause health problems and our doctors are not
adequately trained in nutrition.

Environmental toxins are another major cause of health problems.
Currently medical doctors do not seem to know this and they know little
or nothing about treatments to detoxify.

Curing almost any illness is relatively simple when you already know
THE CAUSE, but we use mostly drugs that do not treat the cause. What
do you think of a medical doctor who recommends a treatment without
knowing the cause of your ailment?

One major problem we have regarding the cause of illness is that most
doctors make little or no attempt to determine the cause. I'm one living
example. I had to learn the cause of my illness in order to save my own life.
I DID THAT. I am living proof that I know the cause of ALS. Now let me
tell you just how simple it is using only logic and reason and no microscope,
clinical study, or anything else. There are about 80 incurable illnesses and
about half of them are neuro degenerative illnesses. Everyone knows that
thousands of us are dying every year from toxic pollution in our air, water
and food. In spite of that, very few doctors ever determine the cause of a
patient's illness BEFORE he dies.

If I was a doctor, and my patient had any one of the 40 or more neuro
illnesses, my very first thought would be a neuro toxin. You don't have to
go to med school to know that a neuro illness could be caused by a neuro
toxin. I believe all these neuro illnesses result eventually in muscle paralysis
and eventually death from that. A neuro toxin can and will cause muscle
paralysis. That's so simple to me that every time I think about it, it makes
me sick that so many people are dying and our medical system does not

understand. In addition to that, the FDA approves many toxic food additives every week, the dentists continue to put toxic Mercury in our fillings, the food companies continue to add MSG to their products, the soft drink companies continue to add Aspartame to their drinks, and on and on. Let me say it another way. The word "toxin" has limited impact but it is synonymous to poison. What if I said the FDA approved adding poison to our food, the dentists add poison to our fillings, our city adds poison to our water supply and our industry adds poison to our air? All that is bad enough, but our government seems to ignore most of that. Our elected officials also ignore the fact that prescription drugs are poison and kill thousands every year while rarely offering a cure.

WAKE UP WASHINGTON. THEY'RE KILLING US. Time for some action.

Solution

Here are several recommendations. If all of these were followed, the result could be a 50% or more drop in the cost of medical care. The first one is the most important. Just imagine, if we had an inexpensive cure for heart disease and cancer, how that would affect our health problems. Of course, that would be devastating for the drug companies, the medical doctors, the pharmacists, etc.

Group medical insurance provides no benefit to the patient and includes many problems. It would be far better for each person to buy their own individual policy which would be guaranteed for their lifetime.

Eliminate MSG as a food additive. It is TOXIC and causes thousands of people health problems. Read the book "Excitotoxins: The Taste That Kills" by Russell L. Blaylock, MD.

Make it illegal for any dentist to use any Mercury dental fillings. Mercury is a neuro toxin and causes many neuro illnesses. Toxin means poison. Why do we allow them to put poison in our teeth?

Begin teaching our children in public schools about nutrition, but mostly the need to avoid non-nutritional foods.

Make this book required reading for all twelfth graders.

REQUIRE OUR MEDICAL SCHOOLS TO TRAIN OUR MEDICAL DOCTORS IN NUTRITION AND IN TREATMENTS TO DETOXIFY.

We need to change the law to allow more freedom of speech about food and dietary supplements.

Establish a department to oversee the FDA and all other government agencies to make sure they are not violating the Constitution. Actually, if I were King, I would terminate anyone in the FDA who has accepted money from Big Pharma.

Establish another department in charge of investigating possible medical cures.

We need an inexpensive way for the FDA to approve natural cures.

It might be a good idea to limit the number of lobbyists from Big Pharma.

It also might be a grand idea to provide some sort of a penalty for BRIBERY, especially where our health is concerned.

Require all medical doctors to read this book and all the books listed in Chapter 4.

If we did all of the above, this would be a real boon to society. It might also solve the illegal immigrant problem. You see, all the displaced people formerly working in the medical field would all be picking crops and there would be no work available for the immigrant.

One final thought and maybe this is even more important than all of the rest. I have thought long and hard about this and decided that our PROFIT-DRIVEN medical care system must be changed. We simply must RESTORE "Freedom of Speech" by allowing providers of natural treatments and natural substances to freely communicate the benefits of their product or treatment. We must take away the almost exclusive use of the word "cure" from the drug companies. Why, because they have proven most of their drugs don't cure. Also, their television advertising should be better controlled or maybe even eliminated, just like we have done to the tobacco companies.

Although HMO's provide lower costs, the patients are not provided the same level of treatment. HMO's should be outlawed. The patient and the doctor should determine the treatment and not the insurance company.

Message for Congress

Here is a list of major events in our history which have been ignored by Congress. Each of you may want to review them because I believe it's time for you to take some action.

1776—The writers of the Constitution chose to ignore Dr. Benjamin Rush when he recommended providing more freedom of medicine.

1841—Congress totally ignored Dr. Ignas Semmelweis when he attempted to have doctors wash their hands to prevent thousands of deaths from infections and was driven to insanity by the medical profession.

1868—Medical Dr. Peter Busch discovered that cancer cannot tolerate a fever or high temperatures. This is another possible cancer cure that has been ignored for over 100 years. This is one of the treatments they use now in Germany.

1934—Dr. Otto Warburg discovered a cure for cancer. This was totally ignored by Congress when the medical profession failed to incorporate Dr. Warburg's discovery in cancer treatment.

1946—Dr. Max Gerson developed a treatment to cure cancer by primarily eating the right foods. In 1945, he brought five cancer patients to Congress to testify about the cancer cure. Congress totally ignored this and today thousands continue to die from cancer and we do not have a cure.

1998—Dr. Louis Ignarro was awarded a Nobel Prize in Medicine for his discovery that Nitric Oxide may prevent and cure many diseases including heart disease. It appears that this valuable discovery has also been ignored.

2002—An article appeared in JAMA which stated clearly that cancer could be reversed with calcium. Again, this was ignored by our medical doctors.

All these events should lead you to conclude that we have a serious problem with our medical system in this country. It appears to be as though we are totally ignoring treatments that may prevent and cure. Rather, our doctors choose to use prescription drugs which rarely cure. Let me remind you of some of the facts in this book:

Thousands of people die every year from drugs. Thousands more die because of our failure to provide cures which we know already exist.

HOW LONG CAN YOU MEMBERS OF CONGRESS GO ON IGNORING ALL THIS? I believe now that it's having disastrous effects on OUR ECONOMY, perhaps it's time for action.

CHAPTER 18

MEDICAL INSURANCE

Medical insurance should only be available with a high deductible such as $2,000 or $3,000 or more. Insurance is only economically feasible when the loss is unexpected. However, most people expect to have up to $2,000 per year in normal medical expenses year in and year out.

This violates one of the main principles of insurance. Insurance will only work effectively when the chance of loss is fortuitous; meaning accidental or unexpected. With so many people in this country having chronic illnesses, medical expenses are certainly not unexpected. The only question is how much will be the cost. No doubt the majority of families will have $2,000 or $3,000 a year in medical expenses year in and year out. If we try to transfer this expense to the insurance companies, we just shoot ourselves in the foot.

Out of every dollar paid for medical insurance, there are administrative costs. These costs for most lines of insurance run around 35%. To put it another way, if you spend $2,000 a year for medical treatments and you wish to transfer that to an insurance company, it will cost you about 50% more or around $3,000 a year. So, let me repeat, looking for insurance for an expected event is unwise.

My conclusion is that medical insurance can only be feasible with a large deductible such as $2,000 a year or higher; maybe even $5000 would be better. This would lower the cost of health insurance remarkably.

It might be wise to have a separate deductible for sickness and for accidental injury. You might have a $200 to $500 deductible for accidental injuries and a $2,000 or higher deductible for sickness.

Another factor is human nature. Some people run to their MD every time they cut their finger or have a runny nose. If it's free, why not? A co-insurance requirement should be mandatory, with a larger amount in the beginning and reducing as the medical costs increase during the year.

Here is one more suggestion for consideration. If the patient has to pay out of his own pocket, that will result in fewer treatments. I think it would be a good idea to have a large deductible like maybe $5,000 a year per person and then a tax benefit or tax credit for amounts less than the deductible. This way the patient will have to pay up front, but would be reimbursed.

People who are reckless with their health should pay higher premiums for their medical insurance than those who are more health minded. Smokers and overweight people should pay higher premiums. A proper rate structure would also encourage people to be healthier.

Now there is a big, big problem with health insurance that demands correction.

It is perfectly legal for a medical insurance company to cancel a person's insurance policy when the person gets really, really sick or develops a terminal illness like I did. What, you can't believe that? Let me tell you how it works.

Let's say that you work 20 or 30 years for a corporation who provides you with medical insurance through a group policy. Then, you get so sick you cannot work any longer. You are forced to quit your job and, by doing so, your medical insurance is terminated. IF you are age 65, then you qualify for Medicare. BUT, if you are not age 65, then you may qualify for insurance but only for a limited length of time and usually at a much higher premium. When this limited insurance runs out, you are left high and dry. You're still sick, unable to work, without medical insurance, and you cannot buy it.

Now that, to my way of thinking, IS A GROSS INJUSTICE.

Congress passed a bill several years ago called 'COBRA.' However, it did not go nearly far enough to fully correct the problem. It was a step in the right direction or maybe a stumble. We need to do more.

Your employer's group medical insurance company receives your premium for many years and now they just turn you loose. I think that insurance companies providing group medical insurance should be required to offer you continuous protection for the rest of your life AND at a fair premium.

CHAPTER 19

INVESTMENT ADVICE

Normally I do not offer investment advice. However, I will make an exception in this case. I'm an investor in common stocks. I suggest caution in buying a stock of any pharmaceutical company for two reasons:

Reason #1

Big Pharma spends twice as much on promotion than they spend on research and development. TWICE AS MUCH ON PROMOTION AS ON RESEARCH. Did you hear an echo?

When a company spends more money on marketing than on producing their product, it usually means they have an inferior product. That should also make you question the integrity of the company

Reason #2

The pharmaceutical companies have been the darlings of Wall Street for several decades. I predict their bubble is about to burst. All the evidence indicates that they are near a saturation point with new drugs. Plus, sooner or later, people will get wise to what's going on. I predict that someday, in the not too distant future, there will be fewer drug companies. When that happens, you surely do not want to be holding any of their stocks in your portfolio. There will be a day of reckoning.

AS AN INVESTOR I INTEND TO NEVER BUY STOCK IN ANY PHARMACEUTICAL COMPANY.

CHAPTER 20

CONCLUSION

At this point I would like to remind you of a few things:

Most drugs do not cure.
Most drugs do not treat the cause.
Most doctors prescribe drugs excessively.
The cost of our present medical system is enormous and it is ineffective.
Something must be done to stop this juggernaut.

Our plan is to mail a copy of this book to each member of Congress plus President Obama and a few more in Washington, DC.

If you agree that we have a problem with our medical system, would you PLEASE consider helping Glenna and I and all our countrymen with our cause. Please write your Senator and Rep in the House of Representatives. The only way this problem will ever be corrected is by government intervention brought about by you and me. Remember, apathy is our common enemy.

Our mission is to have one copy of this book in every home and in the hands of those people who make critical decisions about our health care.

*   *   *

You may want to write your Congress person and here is a sample of what you might say:

Honorable (name of Congress person):

Our medical system in this country is broken and in need of repair plus it is far too expensive.

We urge you to not expand our health care system until you fix it.

You must read the book "Surviving Without Your MD" by Eric and Glenna Edney because it lays out the cold, hard facts causing the problem, plus many suggestions for correcting the problem.

Government intervention is the only chance we have to solve this problem.

Would you please read the book. A book may have already been mailed to you.

John Doe

*   *   *

Here is how you may find your Congress person to whom to write:-

Go to your computer and do a "Search" for USCongress.
Select Congress.org Home
Enter your zip code in the left-hand column "My Elected Officials."
That will provide you with your Congress person by name, also their mailing address and their FAX number.

DO IT NOW. Write your Congress person. Don't procrastinate.
I had planned on writing a book about procrastination, but I never got around to it. Ha-ha-ha
That's why I say again DO IT NOW.

*   *   *

Here's to your good health. We wish you well and pray that you will live a long, healthy life. We hope this book helps you achieve that.

Eric and Glenna Edney

P. S. If you like this book and you agree with it, would you please help us out by telling two or more other people about it and urge them to read it. We strongly believe that everyone should know about what's in this book. Here is one more thought. If you know someone with a serious illness, they might benefit from this book. You might buy one for them or let them read yours.

Web site for Gallstones pg 17

Asthma – & Comfrey root pg. 22

Psoriasis – Airoil – Tar oil – pg 23

Glyconutrients for eyes pg. 25

Boric Acid for eye wash. pg 25

Lipton Tea causing arthritis ? pg 21

Diarrhea & AND FLAGYL prescryption
                                pg. 28 – 35

Toxins cause Cancer pg 55

* Hydrogen Peroxide – pg 56 OR ~~Hydrogen~~ CHLORINE per-
                                                    OXIDE

* Cancer cannot survive pg 57

Cancer Test (Do it yourself for
$165.00 with web site pg 60
        More about cancer book tho
        another web site page 60

RESVERATOL – PG 62

ASPARAGUS CURE – PG 62 – 63

  Codeine / Tylynol pg 66 (combined pill)

The TOXIC DRUG to prevent Cervical Cancer
        * Scary *   PG 88

Swine Flu Influenca – a Hoax pg 90

No evidence of Cholesteral cause heart
        attacks or strokes pg 93

* ED+A & Chelation !! pg 94 – 97 – 98

* Chlorine Dioxide pG 98 – 99 – for Staph

ALS – Caused by Mercury pg 120